Instructor's Manual and Testbank to Accompany

Med-Math

DOSAGE CALCULATION, PREPARATION, AND ADMINISTRATION

FOURTH EDITION

Instructor's Manual and Testbank to Accompany

Henke's Med-Math

DOSAGE CALCULATION, PREPARATION, AND ADMINISTRATION

FOURTH EDITION

Susan Buchholz, RN, BSN, MSN

Assistant Professor
Nursing Department
Georgia Perimeter College
Clarkston, Georgia

LIPPINCOTT WILLIAMS & WILKINS
A **Wolters Kluwer** Company

Philadelphia · Baltimore · New York · London
Buenos Aires · Hong Kong · Sydney · Tokyo

Managing Editor: Doris S. Wray
Acquisition Editor: Margaret Zuccarini

Fourth Edition
Copyright © 2003 by Lippincott Williams & Wilkins.

Copyright © 1999 by Lippincott Williams & Wilkins. All rights reserved. No part of this book may be used or reproduced in any manner whatsoever without written permission with the following exception: testing materials may be copied for classroom use, provided the instructor has adopted its accompanying text, *Henke's Med-Math: Dosage Calculation, Preparation, and Administration,* fourth edition, by Susan Buchholz. Printed in the United States of America. For information, write Lippincott Williams & Wilkins, 530 Walnut Street, Philadelphia, Pennsylvania 19106-3780.

ISBN: 0-7817-4028-2

Any procedure or practice described in this book should be applied by the health care practitioner under appropriate supervision in accordance with professional standards of care used with regard to the unique circumstances that apply in each practice situation. Care has been taken to confirm the accuracy of information presented and to describe generally accepted practices. However, the author, editors, and publisher cannot accept any responsibility for errors or omissions or for any consequences from application of the information in this book and make no warranty, express or implied, with respect to the contents of the book.

Introduction

As I thought about what to put into the *Instructor's Manual and Testbank to Accompany Henke's Med-Math,* I tried to think of what information from other instructor manuals helped me in my teaching. I must confess that sometimes I only used the instructor's manual for the test banks! However, I occasionally used ideas from the manual to be creative in teaching, to try some different things, and to be sure I understood what was the "necessary" content. I tried to do the same with this manual. There is an overview of each chapter from *Med-Math,* suggestions for teaching the content, and a summing up of the basics from the chapter. I hope it helps you as you teach.

Oh yes, there is a test bank, too. There are two pretests you can use for determining the student's basic arithmetic skills; several tests for various chapters; two cumulative dosage tests; and a Med-Math cumulative test. A CD-ROM is included in the Med-Math textbook. This has a 40-question pre-test and 110 questions taken from Chapters 6 to 10.

I have included a pocket card that I make for nursing students. I copy this onto heavier or colored paper. I then laminate these with laminated paper (from an office supply store or they can do it for you) and give them to the nursing students to carry in the clinical setting. There are two pages (found on pages 81 and 82); you can copy one page to the front and one page to the back. Each sheet makes four cards. (I call these "The All-in-One Pocket Cards" or "TAPocketCards" for short.)

Here are some web sites that are useful for finding drug information:

http://www.nursespdr.com/
http://www.rxlist.com/
http://www.pdr.net/

This is a useful site for Palm Pilot/HandSpring users. You can download drug information to your PDA:

http://www.epocrates.com/

Here are two sites that deal with dosage calculations:

Courtesy of John Miller, Tacoma Community College Nursing Program:

http://www.tacoma.ctc.edu/home/jmiller/doscalc.htm

Courtesy of Richard Lakeman:

http://www.geocities.com/HotSprings/8517/Quiz/quiz.htm

Appendix A includes the "answers" to Test Your Clinical Savvy. (These are at the end of Chapters 7, 8, 10, 11, 12, and 13 in the textbook.) Test Your Clinical Savvy was designed to suggest clinical situations where dosage calculations may not have a "right or wrong" solution. Certainly, the math involved in calculations is either correct or incorrect. As an instructor you are encouraged to use these situations to promote critical thinking and get your students to think about several possibilities or options in a clinical setting. Sometimes more information is needed to answer these problems. You may have been in clinical situations where the "answer" is different from the ones included in Appendix A. You are encouraged to discuss these situations with students so that they can see a solution from a different perspective.

Enjoy the wonderful world of calculations!

Susan Buchholz

Contents

CHAPTER 1

Arithmetic Needed for Dosage

Overview of the Chapter

Chapter 1 covers basic arithmetic, and should be a review for a college nursing student. Many people had basic math, but it may have been many years since they studied it. It is important to identify students with problems in calculation and to correct deficiencies before beginning dosage calculations. Material in Chapter 1 includes:

- Multiplying and dividing whole numbers
- Multiplying and dividing fractions
- Decimals
- Percent
- Ratio and proportion

■ Suggestions/Strategies for Teaching

- Assign Chapter 1. Use Test A or Test B in the *Instructor's Manual* (page 21 or 23) as a pre-test or post-test. Use the self-test and proficiency test in *Med-Math* for testing or review.

- Have the students hand work all the problems. Discourage the use of a calculator. If the student cannot do the problems by hand, then there is no guarantee the numbers will be entered correctly in a calculator. Review of the multiplication tables and division (pp. 2 and 3) may be needed.

- Decimals must be thoroughly understood. The metric system is based on decimals. Reading decimals incorrectly can lead to medication errors. A zero should be placed before decimals not preceded by a whole number.

    EXAMPLE: ".5" should be written and said: "0.5"

- Fractions and percents also must be thoroughly understood. Container labels with solution percent can be shown and labels from IV fluids, such as 0.33 NS, 0.9% NaCl, 5% dextrose.

- Changing from decimals to fractions to percent, and back again, should be practiced until the students can do this without mistakes.

- Ratio and proportion and how it relates to dosage calculations is explained in this chapter. The formula method is shown starting in Chapter 6. Both methods are used in *Med-Math*.

- Math review books are available from all major publishing companies. Computer software is also available. If the student has any problems with arithmetic, these resources are suggested. Here are a few web sites that have basic math help.
    - http://school.discovery.com/homeworkhelp/webmath/
        Basic help with all math problems

- http://mathforum.org/library/topics/multiplication/
  Help with multiplication
- http://mathforum.org/library/topics/division
  Help with division
- http://www.aaamath.com/fra.html/
  Although a K–8 site, it thoroughly covers fractions
- http://www.aaamath.com/dec.html
  Although a K–8 site, it thoroughly covers decimals
- http://www.aaamath.com/pct.html
  Although a K–8 site, it thoroughly covers percents

Copyright © 2003 Lippincott Williams & Wilkins, *Instructor's Manual and Testbank to Accompany Henke's Med-Math: Dosage Calculation, Preparation, and Administration,* fourth edition, by Susan Buchholz.

Interpreting the Language of Prescriptions

Overview of the Chapter

Chapter 2 discusses terms used in medication prescription and administration, including:
- Time abbreviations
- Administration routes
- Metric, SI, apothecary, and household abbreviations

■ Suggestions/Strategies for Teaching

- It is an incentive for students to know that once they learn the abbreviations in this chapter, they can interpret any prescription order. Use overhead transparencies or Powerpoint to show medication orders.

- Sample times are given for time abbreviations. These vary in different institutions and different patient/client settings.

- Discussion of times of administration provide an opportunity to introduce the concept of pharmacokinetics (eg, why one drug is ordered bid while another is ordered q4h).

- Latin terms are included to show how the abbreviation is derived. There is no need for the student to memorize them.

- Some commonly accepted abbreviations (eg, "FYI" and "ASAP") can be introduced.

- Use a medication administration record (MAR) to show students how drug orders are handled. Overhead transparencies or Powerpoint can illustrate this, too.

- Show the difference between IV and IVPB by using IV solutions or an overhead transparency.

- Show (or have the students show) household containers and how the measurements compare. As a good demonstration, have the students measure ounces and pour into medication cups marked with "cc" to show the conversions; have them use a teaspoon and a syringe to show the conversion between these; and so on.

- Have the students demonstrate on themselves or others route abbreviations and where they are. Be sure they are accurate regarding OD, OS, and OU.

- The term "prn" is an excellent way to introduce the nursing process and show how a nurse exercises judgment. Example: a postoperative patient is ordered Tylenol PO 650 mg q4h prn; and Morphine Sulfate 4 mg IM q3h prn. Which drug would you use? How would you assess the pain? How often can you give the medications, and how would you know which medication to give the next time the patient has pain?

Copyright © 2003 Lippincott Williams & Wilkins, *Instructor's Manual and Testbank to Accompany Henke's Med-Math: Dosage Calculation, Preparation, and Administration,* fourth edition, by Susan Buchholz.

- Have the students identify discrepancies in orders that are missing one or more of the seven elements of an order. Use medication records, doctor's order sheets, or make up your own! The seven elements:
  - Patient's name
  - Date
  - Time of administration
  - Name of drug
  - Route of administration
  - Dose of drug
  - Physician (or other health care practitioner) name
- Include several orders that are difficult to understand or read. Emphasize that the nurse must not carry out an order that is unclear and must clarify with the physician (or other health care practitioner) who wrote the order.
- Two tests on abbreviations are found on pages 25 and 27 of this manual.

Copyright © 2003 Lippincott Williams & Wilkins, *Instructor's Manual and Testbank to Accompany Henke's Med-Math: Dosage Calculation, Preparation, and Administration,* fourth edition, by Susan Buchholz.

CHAPTER 3

Drug Labels and Packaging

Overview of the Chapter

- What is included on a drug label
- Drug packaging

■ Suggestions/Strategies for Teaching

- Use sample unit and multidose containers for demonstration with the students. Have the students bring in various containers.
- Use various drug labels to illustrate the differences in labels. Use prescription and OTC; have students bring in any drugs to show the labels.
- Sources for labels: OTC are obtained in drugstores/pharmacies. Ask the pharmacist for any sample labels. Prescription drug labels: have the students bring in any drugs they may have access to. Hospital pharmacies occasionally may supply labels. The best source is to have nurses in a hospital save discarded packaging or vials. Pharmaceutical companies occasionally will supply labels. Addresses can be found in the *PDR*.

Metric, Apothecary, and Household Systems of Measurement

Overview of the Chapter

- Metric solid and liquid measures
- Converting in the metric system
- Apothecary liquid measures
- Household liquid measures
- Metric, apothecary, and household equivalents

■ "The All-in-One Pocket Cards"

Included are two pages (pp. 81 and 82) for you to photocopy onto heavier paper or colored paper. I then laminate these with laminated paper from an office supply store (or you can have them professionally done) and give them to the nursing students. The students can carry them in their pockets, and they are useful as the students learn the various systems. Each sheet makes four cards.

■ Suggestions/Strategies for Teaching

- Students should know conversions within and between measurement systems.
- The quick rules for conversions in the metric system are useful for students:
  - Grams to Milligrams Quick Rule, p. 67
  - Milligrams to Grams Quick Rule, p. 69
  - Milligrams to Micrograms Quick Rule, p. 70
  - Micrograms to Milligrams Quick Rule, p. 71
- Emphasize the care needed in converting decimals. Place a zero before any decimal that is not preceded by a whole number.
- Show medication orders and containers that use liquid metric measurements—IV fluids, antacids, cough medicine.
- The apothecary system is still used in the United States and with some medications. Equivalents to know: 1 dram = 4 mL; 1 minim = 1 gtt. Use a plastic medicine cup and syringe to show these measurements.
- Converting grains to milligrams is not an exact equivalent. However, most texts use the following as the conversion factor:
  - gr i = 60 mg
  - 1 gram = gr 15
  - Specifically with Tylenol and aspirin, the conversion is gr i = 65 mg. This is simple enough that the student can learn both conversions.

 Copyright © 2003 Lippincott Williams & Wilkins, *Instructor's Manual and Testbank to Accompany Henke's Med-Math: Dosage Calculation, Preparation, and Administration*, fourth edition, by Susan Buchholz.

- Roman numerals sometimes are used with apothecary measurements. A quick review may be needed.
- The abbreviation "mcg" may be used instead of "μg," because mcg is safer to interpret when reading drug measurement. A written "μg" can mistakenly be read as "mg."
- Use medicine cups and household containers to show household measurements. Use medicine cups with all three measures (metric, apothecary, household) to show the equivalents among the three systems.
- Students can make flash cards with the equivalents to memorize the measurements.
- Two tests on pages 28 and 29 of this manual can be used.

Copyright © 2003 Lippincott Williams & Wilkins, *Instructor's Manual and Testbank to Accompany Henke's Med-Math: Dosage Calculation, Preparation, and Administration*, fourth edition, by Susan Buchholz.

CHAPTER 5

Drug Preparations and Equipment to Measure Doses

Overview of the Chapter

- Routes of medication
- Equipment to measure doses

■ Suggestions/Strategies for Teaching

- Some important points to emphasize:
  - Suspensions must be shaken before pouring, or the dose will not be accurate.
  - The term "parenteral" is not an injection site; it means "by injection."
  - Ordinarily, capsules should not be opened.
  - Usually, unscored tablets should not be broken; in real life, though, tablets can be broken with a commercial pill cutter.
  - Enteric-coated tablets should not be crushed.
  - Oral liquids must be poured at eye level—emphasize the term "meniscus" (p. 86).
  - All liquids are poured to a line—never estimated. A syringe can be used for liquid medication to ensure correct amount. Injections are drawn up to a marked line on the syringe—never estimated.
  - Rounding rules are permitted if the dosage calculation is not an even number. The nurse must decide the degree of accuracy and use the appropriate syringe. General rounding rules: when the last number is 5, round up to the next number; when the number is 4 or less, drop the number.
  - Try to obtain the following drug preparations. Students can contribute, and drugstore and institutional pharmacists can contribute outdated drugs. Nurses in clinical units can save empty bottles and vials. Explain the preparations and routes:
    - Oral
      - Tablets: unscored, scored, coated, enteric-coated, capsule, extended or sustained release tablets, spansules, sublingual tablets, cough tablets
      - Solutions: syrups, elixirs, fluidextracts, tinctures, solutions, suspensions, magmas, gels, emulsions, powders, aqueous solution

Copyright © 2003 Lippincott Williams & Wilkins, *Instructor's Manual and Testbank to Accompany Henke's Med-Math: Dosage Calculation, Preparation, and Administration,* fourth edition, by Susan Buchholz.

- Topical
  - Aerosol powders and liquids, metered dose inhaler, powders, creams, ointments, pastes, vaginal cream with applicator, vaginal suppository, rectal suppository, disposable enema, transdermal medications
- Parenteral
  - IV fluids, single and multidose vials, ampules, parenteral powder
- Demonstrate equipment to administer medication. For this chapter, medication cups, syringes (preferably without a needle), Tubex, and Carpuject can be shown.
- As the students view the preparations and equipment, use a handout to fill in. It provides a focus and a goal. Include trade and generic names, pros and cons to using the specific preparation, precautions in administration, and safety rules.

Copyright © 2003 Lippincott Williams & Wilkins, *Instructor's Manual and Testbank to Accompany Henke's Med-Math: Dosage Calculation, Preparation, and Administration,* fourth edition, by Susan Buchholz.

Calculation of Oral Medications—Solids and Liquids

Overview of the Chapter

- Formula method, ratio proportion method
- Oral solid and liquid calculations

■ Suggestions/Strategies for Teaching

- Explain or review the ratio–proportion method. Introduce or review the formula method. Chapter 6 explains how the formula method is derived, and that it does skip a step in calculation, thereby lessening the possibility of errors. Either method will work, and what is important is that the student get comfortable with one method and stick to it.

- Dimensional analysis is mentioned as a third method for dosage calculations. A simple explanation is included in *Med-Math*, Appendix A. *Clinical Calculations Made Easy,* by Gloria Craig, published by Lippincott, is an excellent book that teaches dimensional analysis.

- Review how to clear decimals (p. 105). Review the quick rules for converting mg, g, and mcg within the metric system.

- Discourage the use of calculators at present. What is most important is setting up the problem with the right data in the right place in order to solve the calculation.

- Repetition is a key to learning math and calculations. Four self-tests are included in this chapter, and three proficiency tests. The CD-ROM has 25 questions from this chapter. Other computer software on dosage calculations can be used.

- Provide a "hands-on" experience using discarded drug labels and drug containers. Students can handle medications and compute doses. Drug orders can be written, and the student must locate the correct drug and compute the answer.

- Students also can practice pouring oral solids and liquids and role play administering them to one another.

- Point out that oral liquid problems use the same calculation method(s) as oral solids. The only differences are that the stock varies and the answer is the number of mL to give.

- Part Two in this manual has four tests on pages 30, 31, 32, and 34.

Copyright © 2003 Lippincott Williams & Wilkins, *Instructor's Manual and Testbank to Accompany Henke's Med-Math: Dosage Calculation, Preparation, and Administration,* fourth edition, by Susan Buchholz.

Liquids for Injection

Overview of the Chapter

- Calculation of liquid injections
- Use of 1-cc and 3-cc syringes
- Calculation of liquid injections using stock medications ordered as ratio or percent
- Insulin injections

■ Suggestions/Strategies for Teaching

- Injection from liquid problems are solved using the same rules as oral solids and liquids. These medications are sterile, and sterile technique is used in preparing and administering them.
- The formula method or ratio–proportion method can be used to solve these calculations. Emphasize that the student get comfortable with one method, and stay with that method for all calculations.
- Show 1-cc and 3-cc syringes and note the markings. Also use an overhead of the syringes, and ask the students to identify the value of each line.
- Provide a lab experience for students to solve problems from discarded or outdated ampules and vials containing liquid. Use 1-cc, 3-cc, and insulin syringes, and have the students calculate and draw up the medication. Use safety precautions with the needles, unless you have a needleless system and needleless vials. Drug companies may also supply empty sterile vials, Tubex holders, and empty containers. You can reuse these by refilling them with water or saline.
- The exactness of the answer depends on the syringe used. The 3-cc syringe uses an answer rounded to the nearest tenth; with the 1-cc syringe, the answer is rounded to the nearest hundredth.
- Minims are marked on the syringes, point out that the minim is an apothecary measure and the marks are not used. Be sure the student understands this, and does not mistake the minim mark for mL.
- Review types of insulin, insulin orders, and preparing two insulins in the same syringe. You may also use sliding scale formulas and Accu-Check formulas to show the students how insulin dose is calculated.
- Emphasize the dose of insulin must be accurate. The 1-cc insulin syringe has 2 Units per line. On the low-dose insulin syringe, each line equals 1 Unit. Any dose up to 50 Units can be drawn up on the low-dose syringe. Some hospitals also have syringes marked in 30 Units that can be used for lower doses.

- Stock medications that are provided in doses of ratio and percent may be difficult to understand. Review concepts in Chapter 1 of converting from percent to decimals to fractions to ratios and back. Two medications that use ratio and percent are Epinephrine 1:1000 and calcium gluconate 10%. Use these as examples to practice.

- Part Two in this manual has two tests on pages 35 and 37. The CD-ROM has 25 questions from this chapter.

Copyright © 2003 Lippincott Williams & Wilkins, *Instructor's Manual and Testbank to Accompany Henke's Med-Math: Dosage Calculation, Preparation, and Administration,* fourth edition, by Susan Buchholz.

Injections From Powders

Overview of the Chapter

- Information about injections from powders
- Application of the formula method and ratio–proportion method to calculate dosages using reconstituted powders

■ Suggestions/Strategies for Teaching

- Reconstitution of powders by nurses varies from institution to institution. Many hospitals now provide IVPB that use a special reconstitution device, so that no calculation is needed. Hospital pharmacies also reconstitute and pre-mix IVPB. This chapter is shorter because the nurse may rarely reconstitute and calculate these medications. However, the nurse should be familiar with the method.

- Once the drug is reconstituted according to the manufacturer's directions, it then becomes a liquid solution. The formula method or ratio proportion method are then used to calculate the dosage.

- Explain the concept of reconstitution. Students have difficulty understanding that powders increase the volume of fluid added to a vial when they go into solution. This is called displacement.

- The students need only be concerned with two numbers: How much liquid should I add? What solution (concentration) did I make?

- Some students become confused and use the label amount of powder and the volume added rather than the solution made.

  EXAMPLE: Stock is 1 g. Add 2.8 mL NS to make 250 mg/mL. Students will want to use 1 g/2.8 mL rather than 250 mg/mL.

- Check with pharmacies and drug companies for practice vials that contain powder, or for outdated vials. Set up a lab experience with vials of powders and directions. The more problems the students can see, the more comfortable they will be in solving them.

- Show the students the most common diluting fluids for injections from powders: sterile water for injection, bacteriostatic water for injection, and normal saline for injection.

- Part Two in this manual has two tests on pages 39 and 43. The CD-ROM has 10 questions.

Copyright © 2003 Lippincott Williams & Wilkins, *Instructor's Manual and Testbank to Accompany Henke's Med-Math: Dosage Calculation, Preparation, and Administration*, fourth edition, by Susan Buchholz.

Calculation of Basic IV Drip Rates

Overview of the Chapter

- Types of IV fluids
- IV drip factors
- IV infusion pumps
- Calculation of basic IV drip rates
- Choosing an IV infusion set; adding medications to IVs; IVPB calculations; changing to IV drip rate

■ Suggestions/Strategies for Teaching

- Two basic IV formulas:

$$\frac{\text{\# mL ordered}}{\text{\# hr to run}} = \text{mL/hr}$$

$$\frac{\text{\# mL/hr} \times \text{drip factor (TF)}}{\text{\# min}} = \text{gtt/min}$$

- Obtain IV solutions, microdrip (60 gtt = 1 mL) tubing, macrodrip tubing, and an IV pump if possible. Show how the drip chambers differ. Demonstrate to the students how to regulate IV flow, and have them practice. The goal is to deliver a specified amount of IV fluid as evenly as possible over a specified amount of time.

- Illustrate how IV orders can be written in several different ways. Use an overhead transparency or Powerpoint to show this.

- Labels for IV fluids are discussed on page 193. All IV fluids must be labeled.

- Adding medication to IV fluid is calculated using the ratio–proportion method or formula method. Reconstitution of powders is done following directions on the vial or ampule, and dose is calculated using the ratio–proportion method or formula method. Some IVPB use a reconstitution device supplied by the manufacturer.

- IV infusion pumps deliver fluid in mL/hr. Use the rule:

$$\frac{\text{\# mL ordered}}{\text{\# hr to run}} = \text{mL/hr}$$

- Guidelines for determining the rate for IVPB are found in the *PDR*, a nurse's drug reference, or hospital medication administration policies.

- Two tests are provided on pages 47 and 49 of this manual. The CD-ROM has 25 questions on basic IV drip rates.

   Copyright © 2003 Lippincott Williams & Wilkins, *Instructor's Manual and Testbank to Accompany Henke's Med-Math: Dosage Calculation, Preparation, and Administration,* fourth edition, by Susan Buchholz.

Special Types of Intravenous Calculations

Overview of the Chapter

Dosage calculations of:

- Units/hour
- mg/hour; g/hour
- mL/hour
- mg/minute
- mcg/minute; mcg/kg/minute; milliunits/minute
- Calculating dosages based on body surface area (BSA)
- Patient-controlled analgesia (PCA)

■ Suggestions/Strategies for Teaching

- The problems in Chapter 10 are advanced IV calculations. These calculations are used mainly in specialty units, especially critical care. Use your judgment as to how much time to spend teaching these.
- The calculations involve several steps. Show the students how to break down the problem into these steps, and it will be easier for them to understand and solve the problem.
- Common IV problems that most students will encounter: heparin IV (units/hour); insulin IV (units/hour); aminophylline IV (mg/hour).
- The formula method and ratio–proportion method are combined for most of these problems, because some of the rules are unique to these calculations.
- Policies for nurses adding medications to IV fluids vary from institution to institution. Some IV solutions are premixed. The most important thing is to verify how much of the drug is in the IV fluid.
- The rule

$$\frac{\text{\# mL ordered}}{\text{\# hr to run}} = \text{mL/hr}$$

  is used to calculate rates on an infusion pump. Most of the medications in this chapter must be given with an infusion pump.
  - Note that mL/hr = gtt/min when using microdrip (60 gtt = 1 mL) tubing.
- Steps in solving mcg/min problems:
  - Use the rule

$$\frac{\text{mg of drug}}{\text{mL fluid}} = \text{mg/mL}$$

  - Change mg to mcg. This will give you mcg per 1 mL.
  - Substitute 60 gtt for 1 mL.
  - Use the formula method to solve for the rate (S or stock will always be 60).

- Steps in solving mcg/kg/min:
  - Use the above formula for mcg/min problems.
  - The D or desired dose in this formula needs to be determined by the kg—multiply the dose desired by the patient's weight in kg.
  - Use the formula method to then solve for the rate.
- Introduce the concept of BSA in m². Show the nomograms, and remind the students that there is one for adults and older children, and one for younger children and infants. Commercial calculators that can calculate BSA more accurately are gradually replacing these nomograms.
- BSA is used in calculating doses for cancer chemotherapy. The physician who orders oncology drugs, the pharmacist, and the nurse must check the BSA and validate the amount of drug ordered. These are serious medication errors if the dose is not correct. Once the dose is determined, calculating the IV drip is a basic calculation.
- PCA is introduced, and the basics of documentation. Documentation varies greatly among settings and institutions.
- Two tests are found on pages 51 and 53 of this manual. The CD-ROM has 25 questions.

Copyright © 2003 Lippincott Williams & Wilkins, *Instructor's Manual and Testbank to Accompany Henke's Med-Math: Dosage Calculation, Preparation, and Administration,* fourth edition, by Susan Buchholz.

Dosage Problems for Infants and Children

Overview of the Chapter

- Some differences in dosage calculations and administration for children versus adults
- Calculating dosages based on mg/kg and body surface area (BSA)

■ Suggestions/Strategies for Teaching

- Chapter 11 presents a brief overview of pediatric dosages. Most drugs for infants and children are administered as oral liquids or intravenous infusion. Guidelines for medication administration, infusion guidelines, and differences in equipment for infants and children can be found in pediatric texts or other pediatric references.
- Safety is key in the dosages of medications for infants and children.
- A calculator can be used to compute a safe dose range.
- Wide variations in weight, age, and development occur among infants and children. The usual way to guarantee a safe dose is to determine mg/kg body weight. Beginning nursing students need to practice this calculation.
- The ratio–proportion method or the formula method may be used to calculate dosages.
- Two tests are included on pages 55 and 57 of this manual. The CD-ROM has problems using BSA and mg/kg.

Information Basic to Administering Drugs

Overview of the Chapter

- Basic drug knowledge (pp. 268–271)
- Pharmacokinetics (brief explanation of the principles)
- Legal and ethical considerations
- Basics of medication orders
- What is some essential information nurses need to know about drugs? About giving medications? About charting?

■ Suggestions/Strategies for Teaching

- Learn/Review/Refresh the five rights of medication administration. Learn/Review/Refresh the three checks in reading medication labels.
- "The All-in-One Pocket Cards": Included are two pages (pp. 78 and 79) for you to photocopy onto heavier paper or colored paper. I then laminate these with laminated paper from an office supply store (or you can have them professionally done) and give them to the nursing students. The students can carry them in their pockets, and they are useful as the students are learning the various systems. Each sheet makes four cards.
- Pharmacokinetics and pharmacodynamics are covered in more detail in nursing pharmacology texts. You may want to cover the basics, however, so that students will begin to understand drug therapy.
- Legal aspects of medication administration need to be stressed. Medication errors are generally made because the five rights were not followed.
- Ethical principles should guide our actions regarding medication administration. Nurses follow the ANA Code for ethical behavior. Nursing fundamentals textbooks also explain the importance of legal and ethical principles.
- Students have difficulty pronouncing names of drugs, especially the generic names. Many references give the phonetic pronunciation. Review how to use phonetic information. An oral quiz with fabulous prizes would be a fun way to learn and review drug names!
- Students need a nursing drug book in clinical areas. Researching drug information takes practice. Here are a few projects to get them started:
  - Ask what information is provided for each drug.
  - Give a list of drugs and doses, and ask if the doses are safe.
  - Give a list of drugs, and ask for their classes and one sign of effectiveness.
  - Ask for three common side effects from several different classes of drugs.
  - Ask students to explain schedules for controlled substances and pregnancy categories.

Copyright © 2003 Lippincott Williams & Wilkins, *Instructor's Manual and Testbank to Accompany Henke's Med-Math: Dosage Calculation, Preparation, and Administration,* fourth edition, by Susan Buchholz.

- Give a list of classes of drugs; ask for physiological action and one or two teaching points unique to each class.

- Give one or two case histories and ask questions that require drug research.

- Emphasize patient teaching with medications. The student could write a formal teaching plan. I find the simplest query works best: What would you tell a family member about this drug? What will it do? What are some side effects or adverse effects they need to watch for?

Copyright © 2003 Lippincott Williams & Wilkins, *Instructor's Manual and Testbank to Accompany Henke's Med-Math: Dosage Calculation, Preparation, and Administration*, fourth edition, by Susan Buchholz.

Administration Procedures

Overview of the Chapter
- Universal precautions
- Systems of medication administration
- Routes of administration—includes basics about each route, safety, pictures, and diagrams

■ Suggestions/Strategies for Teaching

- Chapter 13 is intended as a brief overview of medication administration. More detailed information may be found in any nursing fundamentals textbook.
- Review Universal Precautions. (In 1996 the term Standard Precautions replaced Universal Precautions; the two terms are now interchangeable.) The Centers for Disease Control and Prevention (CDC) still recommends this as the best way to prevent the spread of infection.
- Three systems of administration are presented. These vary among clinical settings and institutions. Reinforce that the five rights and three checks are followed regardless of the setting.
- A lab may be set up for students to practice pouring, counting, and administering drugs, and signing for them.
- Demonstrate the method of obtaining medication from vials with liquids, powders, and ampules. Demonstrate the common injection sites. Videos are available from major publishing companies to demonstrate medication administration. *MedPrep*, a CAI from Lippincott, can also be used.
- Utilize skills/procedure check-offs that nursing fundamentals textbooks use to demonstrate proficiency of skills. *Procedure Checklists to Accompany Fundamentals of Nursing*, by Taylor, Lillis, and LeMone, published by Lippincott, is one reference.

 Copyright © 2003 Lippincott Williams & Wilkins, *Instructor's Manual and Testbank to Accompany Henke's Med-Math: Dosage Calculation, Preparation, and Administration,* fourth edition, by Susan Buchholz.

Name _____ Date _____

TEST A

These arithmetic operations are needed to calculate doses. If you have difficulty in any area, study your Med-Math *workbook, Chapter 1.*

1. Multiply.

   a. $\begin{array}{r} 462 \\ \times 37 \\ \hline \end{array}$

   b. $\frac{5}{7} \times \frac{14}{15}$

   c. $\begin{array}{r} 0.46 \\ \times 0.17 \\ \hline \end{array}$

2. Divide. If necessary, report decimals to two places.

   a. $46\overline{)754}$

   b. $5\frac{1}{4} \div \frac{7}{2}$

   c. $0.004\overline{)0.2}$

3. Change to a decimal. If necessary, report decimals to two places.

   a. $\frac{1}{64}$

   b. $\frac{4}{5}$

4. Change to a fraction and reduce to lowest terms.

   a. 0.15

   b. 0.03

5. In each set, which number has the greater value?

   a. _____ 0.6 or 0.128

   b. _____ 0.25 or 0.4

   c. _____ 0.1 or 0.2

   d. _____ 0.125 or 0.25

6. Reduce fractions to their lowest terms as decimals. If necessary, report decimals to two places.

   a. $\frac{1}{8}$

   b. $\frac{9}{40}$

   c. $\frac{1}{7}$

7. Round off decimals as indicated.

   a. nearest tenth   3.539 _____

   b. nearest hundredth   0.3254 _____

   c. nearest thousandth   0.7253 _____

Copyright © 2003 Lippincott Williams & Wilkins, *Instructor's Manual and Testbank to Accompany Henke's Med-Math: Dosage Calculation, Preparation, and Administration,* fourth edition, by Susan Buchholz.

8. a. Change percent to a fraction: $\frac{1}{3}\%$

   b. Change percent to a decimal: 0.9%

9. Solve ratios to determine the value of x.

   a. $\frac{45}{180} = \frac{3}{x}$ **b.** $11 : 121 :: 3 : x$ **c.** $\frac{0.5}{0.125} = \frac{x}{4}$

Copyright © 2003 Lippincott Williams & Wilkins, *Instructor's Manual and Testbank to Accompany Henke's Med-Math: Dosage Calculation, Preparation, and Administration,* fourth edition, by Susan Buchholz.

Name _____ Date _____

TEST B

These arithmetic operations are needed to calculate doses. If you have difficulty in any area, study your Med-Math *workbook, Chapter 1.*

1. Multiply.

   a. 432
      ×86

   b. $\frac{3}{12} \times \frac{6}{10} \times \frac{4}{8}$

   c. 25.04
      ×16.1

2. Divide. If necessary, report decimals to two places.

   a. $65 \overline{)9240}$

   b. $4\frac{7}{12} \div \frac{5}{3}$

   c. $0.025 \overline{)10}$

3. Change to a decimal. If necessary, report decimals to two places.

   a. $\frac{18}{96}$

   b. $\frac{55}{121}$

4. Change to a fraction and reduce to lowest terms.

   a. 0.004

   b. 0.25

5. In each set, which number has the greater value?

   a. _____ 0.25 or 0.4

   b. _____ 0.5 or 0.125

   c. _____ 0.46 or 0.379

   d. _____ 0.15 or 0.25

6. Reduce fractions to their lowest terms as decimals. If necessary, report decimals to two places.

   a. $\frac{1}{12}$

   b. $\frac{3}{20}$

   c. $\frac{2}{9}$

7. Round off decimals as indicated.

   a. nearest tenth   14.638 _____

   b. nearest hundredth   0.0254 _____

   c. nearest thousandth 0.3333 _____

Copyright © 2003 Lippincott Williams & Wilkins, *Instructor's Manual and Testbank to Accompany Henke's Med-Math: Dosage Calculation, Preparation, and Administration,* fourth edition, by Susan Buchholz.

8. a. Change percent to a fraction: $\frac{1}{4}\%$

   b. Change percent to a decimal: $12\frac{1}{2}\%$

9. Solve ratios to determine the value of x.

   a. $\frac{0.4}{1} = \frac{x}{25}$ **b.** $\frac{7}{x} = \frac{21}{15}$ **c.** $\frac{x}{2.6} = \frac{3}{1}$

Copyright © 2003 Lippincott Williams & Wilkins, *Instructor's Manual and Testbank to Accompany Henke's Med-Math: Dosage Calculation, Preparation, and Administration,* fourth edition, by Susan Buchholz.

■ Chapter 2: Medical Abbreviations—Test A

Name _____ Date _____

TEST A

Directions: Write out the meaning of the following abbreviations. Give sample times for items marked with an asterisk.

1. *ac _____

_____

2. OU _____

3. *tiw _____

_____

4. *q4h _____

_____

5. SC _____

6. PO _____

7. *q12h _____

_____

8. *qd _____

_____

9. *tid _____

_____

10. OS _____

11. mg _____

12. *bid _____

_____

13. mEq _____

14. OD _____

15. *qid _____

_____

Copyright © 2003 Lippincott Williams & Wilkins, *Instructor's Manual and Testbank to Accompany Henke's Med-Math: Dosage Calculation, Preparation, and Administration*, fourth edition, by Susan Buchholz.

16. *q8h   _____

_____

17. *q6h   _____

_____

18. tsp   _____

19. IM   _____

20. mL   _____

Copyright © 2003 Lippincott Williams & Wilkins, *Instructor's Manual and Testbank to Accompany Henke's Med-Math: Dosage Calculation, Preparation, and Administration,* fourth edition, by Susan Buchholz.

Name _____ Date _____

TEST B

A. Directions: *Match the abbreviation with its meaning. There are more abbreviations than necessary.*

1. _____ 10 a, 2 p, 6 p   **a.** qd

2. _____ every day   **b.** OS

3. _____ left eye   **c.** ac

     d. tid

4. _____ as needed   **e.** q6h

5. _____ right eye   **f.** prn

6. _____ 10 a, 2 p, 6 p, 10 p   **g.** mEq

     h. OU

7. _____ every 8 hours   **i.** bid

8. _____ 10 a, 6 p   **j.** qid

9. _____ before meals   **k.** q8h

10. _____ both eyes   **l.** OD

B. Directions: *Write out the meaning of the following abbreviations. Give sample times for items marked with an asterisk.*

1. *q4h   _____

          _____

2. *pc   _____

          _____

3. mL   _____

4. *biw   _____

          _____

5. tsp   _____

6. *qod   _____

          _____

7. IM   _____

8. PO   _____

9. mg   _____

10. SL   _____

Copyright © 2003 Lippincott Williams & Wilkins, *Instructor's Manual and Testbank to Accompany Henke's Med-Math: Dosage Calculation, Preparation, and Administration,* fourth edition, by Susan Buchholz.

Name _____ Date _____

TEST A

Directions: Provide equivalents as indicated.

1. Express as mg

   a. 0.25 g   = _____

   b. 0.015 gm = _____

   c. 50 mcg   = _____

   d. 0.03 g = _____

   e. 1 g   = _____

   f. 1 mcg   = _____

2. Express as g

   a. 30 mg = _____

   b. 0.6 mg = _____

   c. 100 mg = _____

   d. 5 mg   = _____

3. Express as mcg

   a. 0.25 mg = _____

   b. 0.125 mg = _____

   c. 0.5 mg   = _____

   d. 0.1 mg   = _____

   e. 0.01 mg = _____

   f. 0.001 mg = _____

4. Fill in the blanks

   a. dram ii = _____ mL

   b. 1 tsp   = _____ cc

   c. 1 cc   = _____ mL

   d. 1 qt   = _____ L

   e. ½ oz   = _____ cc

   f. 1 minim = _____ gtt

   g. 1 oz   = _____ mL

   h. 1 L   = _____ mL

   i. 1 tbsp = _____ cc

Copyright © 2003 Lippincott Williams & Wilkins, *Instructor's Manual and Testbank to Accompany Henke's Med-Math: Dosage Calculation, Preparation, and Administration*, fourth edition, by Susan Buchholz.

■ Chapter 4: Medical Equivalents—Test B

Name _____ Date _____

TEST B

A. Directions: Provide equivalents as indicated.

1. 1000 mg = _____ g

2. 4 mg   = _____ mcg

3. 100 mg   = _____ g

4. 1 liter   = _____ mL

5. 1 tsp   = _____ cc

6. 0.015 g = _____ mg

7. 0.125 mg = _____ mcg

8. 1 cc   = _____ mL

9. 0.2 g   = _____ mg

10. 1 kg   = _____ lb

11. 15 cc   = _____ oz

12. 1 mg   = _____ g

13. 1 g   = _____ mg

14. 1 tbsp   = _____ cc

15. 10 mcg   = _____ mg

16. 3 drams = _____ mL

17. 0.5 mg   = _____ mcg

18. 1 pint   = _____ cc

19. 15 mg   = _____ g

20. 250 mcg = _____ mg

B. Directions: Fill in the letter of the correct equivalent.

1. _____ 0.5 mg   **a.** 500 mcg   **c.** 5 mcg

   b. 50 mcg   **d.** 0.0005 mcg

2. _____ 0.25 g   **a.** 250 mcg   **c.** 25 mg

   b. 250 mg   **d.** 25 mcg

3. _____ 1 dram   **a.** 4 cc   **c.** 15 cc

   b. 5 mL   **d.** 30 mL

4. _____ 1 oz   **a.** 30 mL   **c.** 5 mL

   b. 15 mL   **d.** 1 mL

5. _____ 60 mg   **a.** 6 g   **c.** 0.06 g

   b. 0.6 g   **d.** 0.0006 g

Copyright © 2003 Lippincott Williams & Wilkins, *Instructor's Manual and Testbank to Accompany Henke's Med-Math: Dosage Calculation, Preparation, and Administration,* fourth edition, by Susan Buchholz.

Name _____ Date _____

TEST A

Directions: Determine the amount to be administered. Show all arithmetic.

1. Order: Inderal 0.02 g PO q6h
   Stock: tablets scored 0.01 g

2. Order: Synthroid 0.15 mg PO qd
   Stock: tablets of 300 mcg scored

3. Order: Sumycin 500 mg PO q6h
   Stock: capsules of 0.25 g

4. Order: Zyloprim 250 mg PO qd
   Stock: scored tablets of 100 mg

5. Order: phenobarbital 0.03 g PO q4h
   Stock: scored tablets of 60 mg

6. Order: digoxin 0.5 mg PO qd
   Stock: capsules labeled 0.25 mg

7. Order: Lanoxin 0.125 mg PO qd
   Stock: tablets of 0.25 mg scored

8. Order: Levothroid 100 mcg qd PO
   Stock: scored tablets 0.2 mg

9. Order: furosemide 80 mg PO qd
   Stock: scored tablets 40 mg

10. Order: Vasotec 500 mcg PO qd
    Stock: scored tablets 1 mg

Copyright © 2003 Lippincott Williams & Wilkins, *Instructor's Manual and Testbank to Accompany Henke's Med-Math: Dosage Calculation, Preparation, and Administration,* fourth edition, by Susan Buchholz.

Name _____ Date _____

TEST B

Directions: Determine the amount to be administered, and place the answer on the line. It is not necessary to show arithmetic.

1. Order: 20 mg PO   Stock: 10-mg tablets scored   _____

2. Order: 0.125 mg PO   Stock: 0.25-mg tablets scored   _____

3. Order: 0.25 mg PO   Stock: 0.125-mg tablets scored   _____

4. Order: 0.5 mg PO   Stock: 0.25-mg tablets scored   _____

5. Order: 250 mg PO   Stock: 0.5-g tablets scored   _____

6. Order: 0.2 g PO   Stock: 400-mg tablets scored   _____

7. Order: 200 mcg PO   Stock: 0.1-mg tablets scored   _____

8. Order: 1 g PO   Stock: 500-mg capsules   _____

9. Order: 200,000 Units/PO   Stock: 100,000-Unit tablets scored   _____

10. Order: 0.01 g PO   Stock: 5-mg tablets scored   _____

11. Order: 0.6 g PO   Stock: 300-mg capsules scored   _____

12. Order: 375 mg PO   Stock: 125-mg capsules   _____

13. Order: 0.3 mg PO   Stock: 600-mcg tablets scored   _____

14. Order: 50 mg PO   Stock: 0.1-g tablets scored   _____

15. Order: 0.1 mg PO   Stock: 100-mcg tablets scored   _____

16. Order: 0.1 g PO   Stock: 100-mg tablets scored   _____

17. Order: 60 mg PO   Stock: 40-mg tablets scored   _____

18. Order: 400 mcg PO   Stock: 0.2-mg tablets scored   _____

19. Order: 0.01 g PO   Stock: 20-mg tablets scored   _____

20. Order: 25 mg PO   Stock: 10-mg tablets scored   _____

Copyright © 2003 Lippincott Williams & Wilkins, *Instructor's Manual and Testbank to Accompany Henke's Med-Math: Dosage Calculation, Preparation, and Administration*, fourth edition, by Susan Buchholz.

Name _____ Date _____

TEST A

Directions: Determine the amount to be administered. Indicate the amount needed on the cup. Show all arithmetic.

1. Order: Dilatin susp. 120 mg PO tid
   Stock: liquid labeled 75 mg per 5 mL

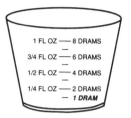

2. Order: digoxin 0.125 mg PO qd
   Stock: bottle of liquid labeled digoxin 0.5 mg per 20 mL

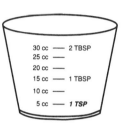

3. Order: tetracycline HCl syrup 0.5 g PO q6h
   Stock: bottle of liquid labeled 250 mg per 10 mL

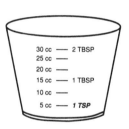

4. Order: Mylanta 30 mL q4h PO prn
   Stock: bottle of liquid labeled Mylanta

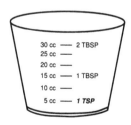

5. Order: Elix. Lanoxin 0.125 mg PO qd
   Stock: liquid labeled 0.25 mg per 10 mL

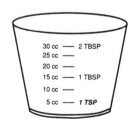

Copyright © 2003 Lippincott Williams & Wilkins, *Instructor's Manual and Testbank to Accompany Henke's Med-Math: Dosage Calculation, Preparation, and Administration,* fourth edition, by Susan Buchholz.

6. Order: Dilatin susp. 100 mg PO tid
   Stock: bottle of liquid labeled 50 mg per 10 mL

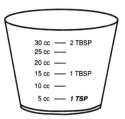

7. Order: Slo-K 20 mEq PO bid
   Stock: bottle of liquid labeled 30 mEq per 15 mL

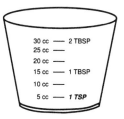

8. Order: Levothroid suspension 100 mcg PO qd
   Stock: bottle of liquid labeled 0.2 mg per 10 mL

9. Order: Bicillin susp. 600,000 Units PO q4h
   Stock: bottle labeled 300,000 Units/5 mL

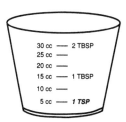

10. Order: promazine HCl 100 mg PO
    Stock: liquid labeled 200 mg/10 mL

Copyright © 2003 Lippincott Williams & Wilkins, *Instructor's Manual and Testbank to Accompany Henke's Med-Math: Dosage Calculation, Preparation, and Administration,* fourth edition, by Susan Buchholz.

Name _____ Date _____

TEST B

Directions: Determine the amount to be administered, and place the answer on the line. It is not necessary to show arithmetic.

1. Order: 20 mg PO   Stock: 10 mg per 4 mL   _____

2. Order: 0.5 g PO   Stock: 250 mg per 6 mL   _____

3. Order: 100 mcg PO   Stock: 0.2 mg per 10 mL   _____

4. Order: 0.1 g PO   Stock: 200 mg per 10 mL   _____

5. Order: 0.25 mg PO   Stock: 0.5 mg per 10 mL   _____

6. Order: 15 mEq PO   Stock: 30 mEq per 40 mL   _____

7. Order: 0.125 mg PO   Stock: 0.5 mg per 20 mL   _____

8. Order: 1 g PO   Stock: 250 mg per 2 mL   _____

9. Order: 500,000 Units PO   Stock: 1,000,000 Units per 20 mL   _____

10. Order: 0.25 mg PO   Stock: 0.5 mg per 5 mL   _____

11. Order: 12 mg PO   Stock: 2 mg per 5 mL   _____

12. Order: 12 mg PO   Stock: 4 mg per 5 mL   _____

13. Order: 500 mg PO   Stock: 0.25 g per 4 mL   _____

14. Order: 160 mg PO   Stock: 40 mg per 5 mL   _____

15. Order: 80 mg PO   Stock: 25 mg per tsp   _____

16. Order: 0.75 g PO   Stock: 250 mg per 5 mL   _____

17. Order: 10 mg PO   Stock: 2 mg per 5 mL   _____

18. Order: 0.25 mg PO   Stock: 0.125 mg per 5 mL   _____

19. Order: 15 mg PO   Stock: 10 mg per 4 mL   _____

20. Order: 0.2 gm PO   Stock: 400 mg per 10 mL   _____

Copyright © 2003 Lippincott Williams & Wilkins, *Instructor's Manual and Testbank to Accompany Henke's Med-Math: Dosage Calculation, Preparation, and Administration*, fourth edition, by Susan Buchholz.

Name _____ Date _____

TEST A

Directions: Determine the volume to be administered. Draw a line on the syringe indicating the amount. Show all arithmetic.

1. Order: Lanoxin 0.125 mg IM 10 A.M.
   Stock: ampule labeled 0.25 mg/2 mL

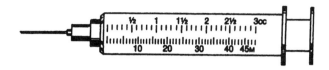

2. Order: penicillin G procaine 600,000
             Units IM q12h
   Stock: vial labeled 500,000 Units/mL

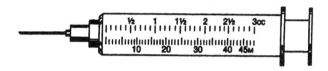

3. Order: morphine sulfate 8 mg SC q4h prn
   Stock: vial labeled 15 mg/mL

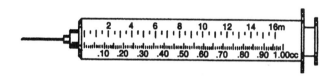

4. Order: 15 Units NPH Humulin insulin SC
   Stock: NPH Humulin 100 Units/mL

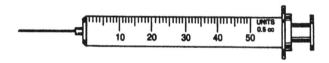

5. Order: diphenhydramine hydrochloride
             40 mg IM stat
   Stock: ampule labeled 50 mg (2-cc size)

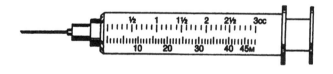

6. Order: levorphanol tartrate 3 mg SC
   Stock: labeled 2 mg/mL

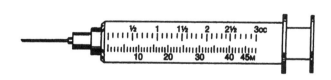

Copyright © 2003 Lippincott Williams & Wilkins, *Instructor's Manual and Testbank to Accompany Henke's Med-Math: Dosage Calculation, Preparation, and Administration,* fourth edition, by Susan Buchholz.

7. Order: epinephrine 0.4 mg SC stat
   Stock: ampule labeled 1:1,000 (2-mL size)

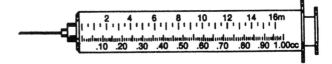

8. Order: magnesium sulfate 500 mg IM
   Stock: ampule labeled 50% (2-mL size)

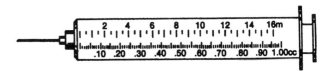

9. Order: Add nitroglycerin 200 mcg to IV stat
   Stock: vial labeled 0.8 mg/mL

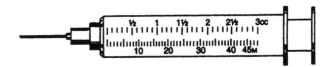

10. Order: oxymorphone HCl 0.75 mg SC
    Stock: vial labeled 1.5 mg/mL

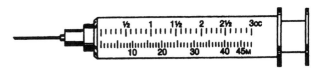

Copyright © 2003 Lippincott Williams & Wilkins, *Instructor's Manual and Testbank to Accompany Henke's Med-Math: Dosage Calculation, Preparation, and Administration,* fourth edition, by Susan Buchholz.

Name _____ Date _____

TEST B

Directions: Determine the volume to be administered. Draw a line on the syringe indicating the amount. Show all arithmetic.

1. Order: cimetadine 225 mg IM stat
   Stock: 300 mg = 2 mL

   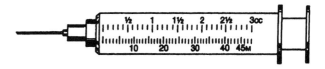

2. Order: gentamycin 60 mg IM q8h
   Stock: 80 mg/2 mL

   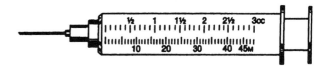

3. Order: heparin sodium 2,000 Units
           SC in abdomen q2h
   Stock: 5,000 Units/mL

   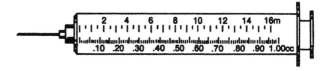

4. Order: Benedryl 25 mg IM stat
   Stock: 50 mg per mL

   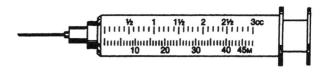

5. Order: caffeine sodium benzoate
           0.25 gm SC stat
   Stock: 0.5 g per 2 mL

   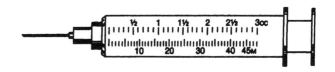

6. Order: Vasoxyl 15 mg IM stat
   Stock: 20 mg in 1 cc

   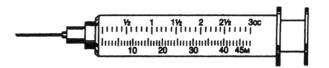

7. Order: Adrenalin 1 mg SC stat
   Stock: ampule labeled 1:1000

   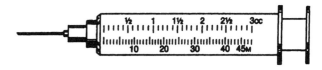

Copyright © 2003 Lippincott Williams & Wilkins, *Instructor's Manual and Testbank to Accompany Henke's Med-Math: Dosage Calculation, Preparation, and Administration,* fourth edition, by Susan Buchholz.

8. Order: furosemide 16 mg IM stat
   Stock: 20 mg/2 mL

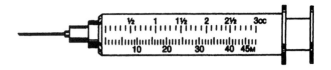

9. Order: Lanoxin 0.25 mg IM stat
   Stock: ampule labeled 0.5 mg/2 mL

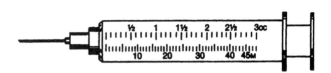

10. Order: morphine sulfate 10 mg SC stat
    Stock: vial labeled 15 mg/mL

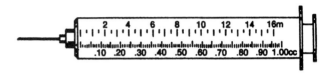

Copyright © 2003 Lippincott Williams & Wilkins, *Instructor's Manual and Testbank to Accompany Henke's Med-Math: Dosage Calculation, Preparation, and Administration,* fourth edition, by Susan Buchholz.

Name _____ Date _____

TEST A

A. *For each problem give the following information:*

Stock powder used   Rule and arithmetic   Label if indicated
Diluting fluid—type and amount   Answer   Storage
Solution and new stock

1. Order: cephradine 250 mg IM q8h
     Stock: vial of powder 250 mg

FIGURE 8-1

IM Dilution Table

Vial Size	Volume of Diluent	Approximate Available Volume	Approximate Available Concentration
250 mg	1.2 mL	1.2 mL	208 mg/mL
500 mg	2.0 mL	2.2 mL	227 mg/mL
1 gram	4.0 mL	4.5 mL	222 mg/mL

For Intramuscular Use: Aseptically add sterile water for injection or bacteriostatic water for injection (containing 0.9% [w/v] benzyl alcohol, or 0.12% methylparaben and 0.014% propylparaben) according to the "IM Dilution Table" above. Intramuscular solutions should be used within 2 hours at room temperature; if stored in the refrigerator at 5°C, solutions retain full potency for 24 hours. Constituted solutions may vary in color from light straw to yellow; however, this does not affect the potency.

2. Order: carbenicillin disodium 0.5 g IM q6h
     Stock: vial of powder 2 grams

FIGURE 8-2

Amount of Diluent to Be Added to the 2-g Vial	Volume to Be Withdrawn for a 1-g Dose
4.0 mL	2.5 mL
5.0 mL	3.0 mL
7.2 mL	4.0 mL

For Intramuscular Use: The 2-g vial should be reconstituted with 4.0 mL of sterile water for injection, 0.5% lidocaine hydrochloride (without epinephrine), or bacteriostatic water containing 0.9% benzyl alcohol. (Preparations containing benzyl alcohol should not be used in neonates.) To facilitate reconstitution, up to 7.2 mL of diluent can be used.

Compatibility and Stability: After reconstitution, no significant loss of potency occurs for up to 24 hours at room temperature, or for 72 hours if refrigerated. Any of these unused solutions should be discarded.

3. Order: ceftazidime (Fortaz) 0.5 IM q8h
  Stock: vial of powder 1 gram

FIGURE 8-3

For Intramuscular Use

Vial Size	Amount of Diluent to Be Added	Approximate Available Volume	Approximate Ceftazidime Concentration
500 mg	1.5 mL	1.8 mL	280 mg/mL
1 gram	3.0 mL	3.6 mL	280 mg/mL

Compatibility and Stability: Ceftazidime, when constituted as directed with sterile water for injection, bacteriostatic water for injection, or 0.5% or 1% lidocaine hydrochloride injection, maintains satisfactory potency for 24 hours at room temperature or for 7 days under refrigeration. Solutions in sterile water for injection that are frozen immediately after constitution in the original containers are stable for 3 months when stored at −20°C. Once thawed, solutions should not be refrozen. Thawed solutions may be stored for up to 8 hours at room temperature or for 4 days in a refrigerator.

---

4. Order: ampicillin sodium 0.5 g IM
  Stock: vial of powder 500 mg

FIGURE 8-4

Label Claim	Recommended Amount of Diluent	Withdrawable Volume	Concentration
500 mg	1.8 mL	2.0 mL	250 mg/mL
1.0 gram	3.4 mL	4.0 mL	250 mg/mL
2.0 gram	6.8 mL	8.0 mL	250 mg/mL

For Intramuscular or Intravenous Use: For dilution of 500-mg, 1-gram, and 2-gram vials, dissolve contents of a vial with the amount of sterile water for injection, USP, or bacteriostatic water for injection, USP, listed in the table above.

Although the 1-gram and 2-gram vials are primarily for intravenous use, they may be administered intramuscularly when the 250-mg or 500-mg vials are unavailable. In such instances, dissolve in 3.4 or 6.8 mL sterile water for injection, USP, to give a final concentration of 250 mg/mL.

Compatibility and Stability: The above solutions must be used within 1 hour after reconstitution.

Copyright © 2003 Lippincott Williams & Wilkins, *Instructor's Manual and Testbank to Accompany Henke's Med-Math: Dosage Calculation, Preparation, and Administration,* fourth edition, by Susan Buchholz.

5. Order: cefotaxime 0.4 g IM q6h
   Stock: vial of powder 1 gram

FIGURE 8-5

Preparation of Cefotaxime

Strength	Diluent (mL)	Withdrawable Volume (mL)	Approximate Concentration
1-g vial (im)	3	3.4	300 mg/mL
2-g vial (im)	5	6.0	330 mg/mL

For Intramuscular Use: Reconstitute vials with sterile water for injection or bacteriostatic water for injection as described above.

Compatibility and Stability: Solutions of Cefotaxime reconstituted as described above maintain satisfactory potency for 24 hours at room temperature (at or below 22°C), for 10 days under refrigeration (at or below 5°C), or for at least 13 weeks frozen.

B. Mental Solutions to Powder Problems

Many powder problems can be answered without written work. Indicate your answers to the following questions with four statements. Storage is not included.

Diluting fluid and amount
Solution and new stock
Answer
Label

1. Order: 400,000 Units IM
   Stock: vial of powder labeled 1 million Units
   Directions: Dissolve with 4.6 mL sterile water for injection to make 200,000 Units/mL.

_____

_____

_____

_____

2. Order: 0.5 gm IM
   Stock: vial of powder labeled 1 gram
   Directions: Add 2.5 mL sterile water for injection to make 1 gram per 3 mL.

_____

_____

_____

_____

Copyright © 2003 Lippincott Williams & Wilkins, *Instructor's Manual and Testbank to Accompany Henke's Med-Math: Dosage Calculation, Preparation, and Administration*, fourth edition, by Susan Buchholz.

3. Order: 150 mg IM
    Stock: ampule of powder labeled 500 mg
    Directions: Add 5 mL sterile water for injection to make 100 mg/mL.

_____

_____

_____

_____

4. Order: 150 mg IM
    Stock: vial of powder labeled 250 mg
    Directions: Add 0.9 mL sterile water for injection to make 250 mg/mL.

_____

_____

_____

_____

5. Order: 0.5 g IM
    Stock: vial of powder labeled 2 grams
    Directions: Add 4 mL sterile water to make a solution of 1 gram = 2.5 mL.

_____

_____

_____

_____

Copyright © 2003 Lippincott Williams & Wilkins, *Instructor's Manual and Testbank to Accompany Henke's Med-Math: Dosage Calculation, Preparation, and Administration,* fourth edition, by Susan Buchholz.

Name _____ Date _____

TEST B

A. *For each problem give the following information:*

Stock powder used   Rule and arithmetic   Label if indicated
Diluting fluid—type and amount   Answer   Storage
Solution and new stock

1. Order: cefoxitin 0.8 g IM q6h
     Stock: vial of powder 1 gram

FIGURE 8-6

Strength	Amount of Diluent to Be Added	Approximate Withdrawable Volume	Approximate Average Concentration
1-gram vial	2 mL (IM)	2.5 mL	400 mg/mL
2-gram vial	4 mL (IM)	5 mL	400 mg/mL
1-gram vial	10 mL (IV)	10.5 mL	95 mg/mL

For Intramuscular or Intravenous Use.

Compatibility and Stability: Cefoxitin, as constituted with sterile water for injection, bacteriostatic water for injection, or 0.5% or 1% lidocaine hydrochloride solution (without epinephrine) maintains satisfactory potency for 24 hours at room temperature, for 1 week under refrigeration (below 5°C), and for at least 30 weeks in the frozen state.

---

2. Order: penicillin G potassium 250,000 Units IM
     Stock: vial of one million Units of powder

FIGURE 8-7

Reconstitution: 1,000,000-Unit vial: Add 9.6 mL, 4.6 mL, or 3.6 mL diluent to provide 100,000 Units, 200,000 Units, or 250,000 Units per mL, respectively.

Storage: The dry powder is relatively stable and may be stored at room temperature without significant loss of potency. Sterile solutions may be kept in the refrigerator for 1 week without significant loss of potency. Solutions prepared for intravenous infusion are stable at room temperature for at least 24 hours.

Copyright © 2003 Lippincott Williams & Wilkins, *Instructor's Manual and Testbank to Accompany Henke's Med-Math: Dosage Calculation, Preparation, and Administration,* fourth edition, by Susan Buchholz.

3. Order: cefazolin 0.4 g IM q8h
    Stock: vial of powder 500 mg

FIGURE 8-8

Single-Dose Vials: For IM injection, IV direct (bolus) injection, or IV infusion, reconstitute with sterile water for injection according to the table below. Shake well.

Vial Size	Amount of Diluent	Approximate Concentration	Approximate Available Volume
500 mg	2.0 mL	225 mg/mL	2.2 mL
1 gram	2.5 mL	330 mg/mL	3.0 mL

Compatibility and Stability: When reconstituted or diluted according to the instructions above, sterile cefazolin sodium is stable for 24 hours at room temperature or for 10 days if stored under refrigeration (5°C or 41°F). Reconstituted solutions may range in color from pale yellow to yellow without a change in potency.

---

4. Order: ticarcillin 0.5 g IM
    Stock: vial of powder 1 gram

FIGURE 8-9

Directions for Use: 1-gram, 3-gram, and 6-gram standard vials.

Intramuscular Use (concentration approximately 385 mg/mL): For initial reconstitution, use sterile water for injection, USP, sodium chloride injection, USP, or 1% lidocaine hydrochloride solution* (without epinephrine).

Each gram of ticarcillin should be reconstituted with 2 mL of sterile water for injection, USP, sodium chloride injection, USP, or 1% lidocaine hydrochloride solution* (without epinephrine) and used promptly. Each 2.6 mL of the resulting solution will then contain 1 g of ticarcillin.

As with all intramuscular preparations, ticarcillin disodium should be injected well within the body of a relatively large muscle, using usual techniques and precautions.

*For full product information, refer to manufacturer's package insert for lidocaine hydrochloride.

Copyright © 2003 Lippincott Williams & Wilkins, *Instructor's Manual and Testbank to Accompany Henke's Med-Math: Dosage Calculation, Preparation, and Administration,* fourth edition, by Susan Buchholz.

5. Order: cefoperazone 380 mg IM q12h
   Stock: vial of powder 2 grams

FIGURE 8-10

Preparations for Intramuscular Injection: Any suitable solution may be used to prepare cefoperazone powder for intramuscular injection. When concentrations of 250 mg/mL or more are to be administered, a lidocaine solution should be used. These solutions should be prepared using a combination of sterile water for injection and 2% lidocaine hydrochloride injection (USP) that approximates a 0.5% lidocaine hydrochloride solution. A two-step dilution process as follows is recommended. First, add the required amount of sterile water for injection, and agitate until Cefobid powder is completely dissolved. Second, add the required amount of 2% lidocaine and mix.

Vial Size	Final Cefoperazone Concentration	Step 1: Volume of Sterile Water	Step 2: Volume of 2% Lidocaine	Withdrawable Volume
1-gram vial	333 mg/mL	2.0 mL	0.6 mL	3 mL
	250 mg/mL	2.8 mL	1.0 mL	4 mL
2-gram vial	333 mg/mL	3.8 mL	1.2 mL	6 mL
	250 mg/mL	5.4 mL	1.8 mL	8 mL

B. Mental Solutions to Powder Problems

Many powder problems can be answered without written work. Indicate your answers to the following questions with four statements. Storage is not included.

Diluting fluid and amount
Solution and new stock
Answer
Label

1. Order: 0.66 g IM
   Stock: vial of powder labeled 1 gram
   Directions: Add 2.5 mL sterile water for injection to make 330 mg/mL.

---

2. Order: 600 mg IM
   Stock: vial of powder labeled 1 gram
   Directions: Add 2 mL sterile water for injection to make 400 mg/mL.

Copyright © 2003 Lippincott Williams & Wilkins, *Instructor's Manual and Testbank to Accompany Henke's Med-Math: Dosage Calculation, Preparation, and Administration,* fourth edition, by Susan Buchholz.

3. Order: 450 mg IM
   Stock: vial of powder labeled 500 mg
   Directions: Add 2 mL sterile water for injection to make 225 mg/mL.

   _____

   _____

   _____

   _____

4. Order: 100 mg IM
   Stock: ampule of powder labeled 250 mg
   Directions: Add 3.8 mL sterile water for injection to make 50 mg/mL.

   _____

   _____

   _____

   _____

5. Order: 150 mg IM
   Stock: vial of powder labeled 250 mg
   Directions: Add 2 mL sterile water to make a solution of 125 mg/mL.

   _____

   _____

   _____

   _____

Copyright © 2003 Lippincott Williams & Wilkins, *Instructor's Manual and Testbank to Accompany Henke's Med-Math: Dosage Calculation, Preparation, and Administration,* fourth edition, by Susan Buchholz.

Name _____ Date _____

TEST A

Directions: Show the formula used for solving the problems and all arithmetic.

1. Order: 1000 mL D5W IV over 16 hr
   Available: microtubing

2. Order: 500 mL ½ NS IV
              run 70 mL/hr on a pump
   How many hours will the IV run?

3. Order: aminophylline 500 mg in 500 mL D5W
              run 50 mL/hr on a pump
   Available: aminophylline comes as an ampule of liquid labeled 1 gram/10 mL

4. Order: doxycycline 100 mg IVPB q8h
   Available: macrotubing 10 gtt/mL

Drug	Diluent	Time
doxycycline	250 mL (100 mg) D5W, NS	1 hr (100 mg)
Vibramycin	500 mL (200 mg) D5W, NS	2 hr (200 mg)

5. Order: 150 mL 5% NaCl over 3 hr

6. Order: vancomycin 500 mg IVPB every 8 hr
   Available: vial of powder labeled 500 mg
              macrotubing 10 gtt/mL

Drug	Diluent	Time
vancomycin	100 mL (500 mg) D5W, NS	1 hr (500 mg)
Vancocin®	250 mL (1 gram) D5W, NS	2 hr (1 gram)

7. Order: 500 mL D5 ⅓ NS IV 4 A.M. to 4 P.M.
   Available: pump

Copyright © 2003 Lippincott Williams & Wilkins, *Instructor's Manual and Testbank to Accompany Henke's Med-Math: Dosage Calculation, Preparation, and Administration*, fourth edition, by Susan Buchholz.

8. Order: 1000 mL D5 S with 20 mEq KCl
                run 150 mL/hr
   Available: KCl comes in a vial of liquid labeled 10 mEq per 4 mL
                no pump; macrotubing 10 gtt/mL
   What tubing will you use?

9. Order: 500 mL D5W IV KVO at 50 mL/hr

10. Order: imipenem–cilastatin 0.5 g IVPB q6h
    Available: macrotubing 10 gtt/mL

Drug	Diluent	Time
imipenem	100 mL (500 mg) D5W, NS	20–30 min
cilastatin	250 mL (1 gram) D5W, NS	40–60 min (500 mg)

Copyright © 2003 Lippincott Williams & Wilkins, *Instructor's Manual and Testbank to Accompany Henke's Med-Math: Dosage Calculation, Preparation, and Administration*, fourth edition, by Susan Buchholz.

Name _____ Date _____

TEST B

Directions: Show the formula used for solving the problems and all arithmetic.

1. Order: 250 mL ½ NS IV
                        run 60 mL/hr on a pump
      How many hours will the IV run?

2. Order: 500 mL D5 NS IV
                        run 60 mL/hr on a pump

3. Order: cefotaxime 1 g IVPB q8h

Drug	Diluent	Time
cefotaxime Claforan	50 mL (1 gram) D5W, NS 100 mL (2 grams) D5W, NS	15–30 min

4. Order: 1000 mL D5W with 30 mEq KCl IV 10 A.M. to 4 P.M.
      Available: KCl comes as a vial of liquid labeled 40 mEq per 20 mL
                          macrotubing 20 gtt/mL

5. Order: 100 mL D5W IV
                        run from 12 midnight to 6 A.M.

6. Order: aminophylline 1 g in 1000 mL D5W IV at 75 mL/hr
                        pump is required
      Available: aminophylline comes as an ampule labeled 1 gram = 10 mL

7. Order: Intralipid 500 mL q6h IV
                        other IV fluid is infusing at 80 mL/hr
      What is the 24-hr parenteral intake?

Copyright © 2003 Lippincott Williams & Wilkins, *Instructor's Manual and Testbank to Accompany Henke's Med-Math: Dosage Calculation, Preparation, and Administration,* fourth edition, by Susan Buchholz.

8. Order: fluconazole 200 mg IVPB qd
                   give over ½ hr
   Available: vial labeled 2 mg/mL
                   macrotubing 10 gtt/mL

9. Order: doxycycline 100 mg IVPB q12h
   Available: vial 100 mg powder
                   macrotubing 10 gtt/mL

Drug	Diluent	Time
doxycycline	250 mL (100 mg) D5W, NS	1 hr (100 mg)
Vibramycin	500 mL (200 mg) D5W, NS	2 hr (200 mg)

10. Order: 500 mL D5 ⅓ NS IV KVO for 24 hr

Copyright © 2003 Lippincott Williams & Wilkins, *Instructor's Manual and Testbank to Accompany Henke's Med-Math: Dosage Calculation, Preparation, and Administration,* fourth edition, by Susan Buchholz.

Name _____ Date _____

TEST A

Directions: Show the formula used for solving the problems and all arithmetic. What is the infusion rate?

1. Order: infuse heparin 1100 Units qh IV
   Available: infusion pump; standard solution of 25,000 Units heparin in 250 mL D5W

2. Order: vasopressin 30 Units/hr IV
   Available: infusion pump; standard solution of 200 Units vasopressin; 500 mL D5W

3. Order: fentanyl 600 mcg/hr IV
   Available: infusion pump; solution concentration of 500 mcg/mL

4. Order: start naloxone at 0.4 mg/hr IV; titrate according to response
   Available: infusion pump; standard solution of 2 mg in 500 mL D5W

5. Order: Levophed 12 mcg/min IV
   Available: infusion pump; standard solution of 4 mg in 250 mL D5W

6. Order: epinephrine drip 2 mcg/min IV
   Available: infusion pump; standard solution of 2 mg in 500 mL D5W

7. Order: metaraminol 30 mcg/min IV
   Available: infusion pump; standard solution of 50 mg in 250 mL NS

8. Order: Isuprel 4 mcg/min IV
   Available: infusion pump; standard solution of 2 mg in 250 mL D5W

9. Order: Pitocin 1 milliunit/min IV
   Available: infusion pump; solution of 20 Units in 1000 mL Ringer's solution

10. Order: Taxol 300 mg in 500 mL D5W (glass bottle) IV over 24 hr
    Available: infusion pump; glass bottle of 500 mL D5W
                 Protocol for Taxol is 175 mg/m². Patient's height 5'8"; weight 145
                 kg; BSA 1.7 m².

    a. Is the order of 300 mg correct?

    b. What is the IV pump infusion rate?

Copyright © 2003 Lippincott Williams & Wilkins, *Instructor's Manual and Testbank to Accompany Henke's Med-Math: Dosage Calculation, Preparation, and Administration,* fourth edition, by Susan Buchholz.

Name _____ Date _____

TEST B

Directions: Show the formula used for solving the problems and all arithmetic. What is the infusion rate?

1. Order: Heparin 1400 Units IV qh
   Available: infusion pump; standard solution of 25,000 Units heparin in 250 mL D5W

2. Order: Pitressin 12 Units/hr IV
   Available: infusion pump; standard solution of 200 Units Pitressin in 500 mL D5W

3. Order: verapamil 1 mg/hr IV
   Available: infusion pump; solution of 10 mg/100 mL D5W

4. Order: norepinephrine 16 mcg/min IV
   Available: infusion pump; standard solution of 4 mg in 250 mL D5W

5. Order: start epinephrine drip at 1 mcg/min
   Available: infusion pump; standard solution of 2 mg in 250 mL D5W

6. Order: Aramine 50 mg IV in 250 mL D5W on a pump; titrate to 60 mcg/min
   Available: infusion pump; solution of 50 mg in 250 mL D5W

7. Order: dobutamine 2.5 mcg/kg/min IV
   Available: infusion pump; standard solution of 500 mg in 250 mL D5W
   Patient's weight 60 kg

8. Order: normodyne 0.5 mg/min IV
   Available: infusion pump; standard solution of 200 mg/200 mL

Copyright © 2003 Lippincott Williams & Wilkins, *Instructor's Manual and Testbank to Accompany Henke's Med-Math: Dosage Calculation, Preparation, and Administration,* fourth edition, by Susan Buchholz.

9. Order: aminophylline 60 mg/hr IV
   Available: infusion pump; standard solution of 250 mg in 250 mL D5W

10. Order: ARA C 170 mg in 1 L D5W over 24 hr
    Available: infusion pump; 1 L of D5W
                Protocol for ARA C is 100 mg/m^2. Patient's height 5'3"; weight
                143 kg; BSA 1.7 m^2.

   a. Is the order of 170 mg correct?

   b. What is the IV pump infusion rate?

Copyright © 2003 Lippincott Williams & Wilkins, *Instructor's Manual and Testbank to Accompany Henke's Med-Math: Dosage Calculation, Preparation, and Administration*, fourth edition, by Susan Buchholz.

Name _____ Date _____

TEST A

1. Order: amoxicillin oral suspension 100 mg PO q8h
   Stock: bottle labeled 125 mg per 5 mL
               Baby weighs 15 kg
               Literature: 20–40 mg/kg/day in divided doses

   a. Is dose safe?

   b. How much would you pour?

2. Order: amantadine HCl 35 mg PO tid
   Stock: bottle labeled 50 mg/5 mL
               3-year-old weighs 35 lb
               Literature: 4.4–8.8 mg/kg/day in three divided doses not to exceed 150 mg/day

   a. Is dose safe?

   b. How much would you pour?

3. Order: acetaminophen liquid 100 mg PO q4h prn for temperature above 101°F
   Stock: Liquid in a dropper bottle labeled 80 mg/0.8 cc
               Dose is safe

   How much would you prepare?

4. Order: Augmentin 40 mg/kg/day = 175 mg PO q8h
   Stock: oral suspension 125 mg/5 mL
               3-year-old weighs 4.3 kg

   How much would you pour?

5. Order: phenobarbital 30 mg IM stat
   Stock: ampule labeled 60 mg/2 mL
               1-year-old weighs 22 lb
               Literature: 3–5 mg/kg

   a. Is dose safe?

   b. How much would you pour?

6. Order: penicillin 6 G benzathine 2.4 MU × 1 dose IM
   Stock: vial 600,000 Units/mL
               17-year-old, 48 kg, with primary syphilis
               Literature: IM 50,000 U/kg in a single dose

   a. Is dose safe?

   b. How much would you pour?

Copyright © 2003 Lippincott Williams & Wilkins, *Instructor's Manual and Testbank to Accompany Henke's Med-Math: Dosage Calculation, Preparation, and Administration*, fourth edition, by Susan Buchholz.

7. Order: gentamycin 10 mg IV q12h in D5 ¼ NS
    Stock: vial gentamycin pediatric 10 mg/mL
                 Infant 4 kg
                 Literature: 2.5 mg/kg q12h
                 Concentration for IVPB is 1 mg/mL

    a. Is dose safe?

    b. What amount would you prepare?

8. Order: D5 ⅓ NS IV + 10 mEq KCl per liter at 35 cc/hr maintenance
    Stock: 1000 mL D5 ⅓ NS; KCl 40 mEq/20 mL in fusion pump; Buretrol used
                 6-year-old weighing 20.5 kg

    a. Calculate the amount of KCl needed.

    b. How would you set the Buretrol?

    c. How would you set the pump?

9. Order: gentamicin 75 mg IVPB q8h
    Stock: vial labeled 40 mg/mL; secondary infusion set 10 gtt/mL; infusion pump
                 17-year-old (follow adult guidelines)
                 Literature: dilute in 100 mL NS; give over 1 hr

    a. How much gentamycin is needed?

    b. What is the IVPB drip rate?

10. Order: vancomycin 100 mg IV q8h in 20 mL D5 ⅓ NS over 30 min
     Stock: vancomycin reconstituted to 500 mg/6 mL; Buretrol; infusion pump
                 1-year-old weighs 15 lb
                 Literature: 44 mg/kg in divided doses; dilute to 5 mg/mL

    a. Is the dose safe? Is the diluent safe?

    b. How would you set the Buretrol?

    c. How would you set the pump?

Copyright © 2003 Lippincott Williams & Wilkins, *Instructor's Manual and Testbank to Accompany Henke's Med-Math: Dosage Calculation, Preparation, and Administration,* fourth edition, by Susan Buchholz.

Name _____ Date _____

TEST B

1. Order: ethambutol 0.6 g PO qd
   Stock: 100-mg scored tablets; 400-mg scored tablets
                14-year-old weighs 90 lb
                Literature: > 13 years: give 15 mg/kg/day

   a. Is dose safe?

   b. What amount would you pour?

2. Order: lanoxin 0.045 mg PO qd
   Stock: liquid in a dropper bottle 0.05 mg/1 cc
                Dose is safe.

   How much would you prepare?

3. Order: Tylenol 80 mg PO q4h prn temp 100.9°F
   Stock: liquid labeled 165 mg/5 mL
                Weight: 8.4 kg
                Literature: recommends 10 mg/kg

   a. Is dose safe?

   b. What amount would you prepare?

4. Order: Slo-Phylline 125 mg PO q8h
   Stock: liquid labeled 80 mg/15 mL
                Weight: 18.9 kg; age: 6 years
                Literature: recommends 5 mg/kg loading dose and 4 mg/kg q6h
                If dose needs to be adjusted for children ages 1–9, do not exceed 24 mg/kg/day

   a. Is dose safe?

   b. What amount would you prepare?

5. Order: cefuroxime 75 mg/kg/day = 210 mg in 20 mL D5 ⅓ NS q8h IVPB over 30 min
   Stock: 750-mg vial of powder; infusion pump (mL/hr); Buretrol
                Weight: 8.4 kg
                Literature: recommends 50–100 mg/kg/day in equally divided doses every 6–8 hr
                Dilute 750 mg IV initially with 10 mL sterile water for injection to provide 90 mg/mL

   a. Is dose safe?

   b. How would you prepare?

Copyright © 2003 Lippincott Williams & Wilkins, *Instructor's Manual and Testbank to Accompany Henke's Med-Math: Dosage Calculation, Preparation, and Administration,* fourth edition, by Susan Buchholz.

6. Order: cefazolin 150 mg IM q8h
   Stock: 500-mg vial of powder; directions say to add 2 mL to make a solution of 225 mg/mL
                Child weighs 20 lb
                Literature: for 20 lb (9 kg), 50 mg/kg/day divided into three doses
                Approximate single dose q8h is 150 mg

   a. Is dose safe?

   b. How much would you prepare?

7. Order: diphenhydramine 15 mg deep IM q6h
   Stock: 50 mg/mL
                3-year-old weighing 12 kg with a drug reaction
                Literature: 5 mg/kg/day in divided doses not to exceed 300 mg/day

   a. Is dose safe?

   b. How much would you prepare?

8. Order: tobramycin 40 mg IVPB D5 ⅓ NS 20 cc q8h
   Stock: vial labeled 80 mg/2 mL; Buretrol; infusion pump
                Child weighs 19 kg; 6 years old
                Literature: 6–7.5 mg/kg/day in three or four equal doses; infuse over 30 min

   a. Is dose safe?

   b. How much would you prepare?
      How would you set this up?

9. Order: cefuroxime 210 mg in 20 mL D5 ⅓ NS q8h
   Stock: 750 mg vial of powder; Buretrol; infusion pump
                Dilute 750 mg initially with 10 mL sterile water for injection to make 90 mg/mL
                Infant weighs 4.8 kg
                Literature: 75 mg/kg/day

   a. Is dose safe?

   b. How much would you prepare?
      How would you set this up?

10. Order: prophylactic penicillin benzathine 1.2 MU q28d IM
    Stock: vial labeled 600,000 Units/mL
                8-year-old, 26 kg with rheumatic fever
                Literature: therapeutic IM dose in 1.2 MU in a single dose q month,
                or 600,000 Units q 2 weeks

    a. Is dose safe?

    b. How much would you prepare?

Copyright © 2003 Lippincott Williams & Wilkins, *Instructor's Manual and Testbank to Accompany Henke's Med-Math: Dosage Calculation, Preparation, and Administration,* fourth edition, by Susan Buchholz.

Name _____ Date _____

TEST A

Directions: Show all work.

1. Order: digoxin 0.5 mg qd
   Stock: scored tablets 0.25 mg

2. Order: elixir of Dimetane 25 mg bid
   Stock: liquid in a bottle labeled 10 mg = 4 mL

3. Order: ascorbic acid 0.1 gm bid
   Stock: scored tablets 200 mg

4. Order: aqueous penicillin 150,000 Units IM q4h
   Stock: vial of powder labeled 1,000,000 Units
   Directions: Add 9.6 mL DW to make 100,000 Units/mL

5. Order: sodium phenobarbital 60 mg IM
   Stock: ampule labeled 120 mg/2 mL

6. Order: imipenem—cilastatin 1 g IVPB q6h
                macrodrip tubing 10 ggt/mL is available

Drug	Diluent	Time
imipenem	100 mL (500 mg) D5W, NS	20–30 min (500 mg)
cilastatin	250 mL (1 gram) D5W, NS	40–60 min (1 gram)
Primaxin®		

7. Order: NPH insulin U 30 qd sc at 7:30 A.M.
   Stock: NPH insulin U 100/mL
                an insulin syringe is available

Provide three statements describing what you would do.

Copyright © 2003 Lippincott Williams & Wilkins, *Instructor's Manual and Testbank to Accompany Henke's Med-Math: Dosage Calculation, Preparation, and Administration,* fourth edition, by Susan Buchholz.

8. Order: 600 mL D5 ½ NS
                 run 150 cc/hr IV
                 macrotubing 10 gtt/mL is available

   a. What are the gtt/min?

   b. How many hours will the IV run?

9. Order: morphine sulfate 8 mg SC stat
   Stock: vial of liquid labeled 15 mg/mL

10. Order: 25,000 U heparin in 250 cc D5W
                 infuse 1500 Units/hr IV
                 an IV pump is available

   What is the drip rate?

Copyright © 2003 Lippincott Williams & Wilkins, *Instructor's Manual and Testbank to Accompany Henke's Med-Math: Dosage Calculation, Preparation, and Administration,* fourth edition, by Susan Buchholz.

Name _____ Date _____

TEST B

Directions: Show all work.

1. Order: digoxin 0.125 mg PO qd
   Stock: bottle of liquid labeled digoxin 0.5 mg per 20 mL

2. Order: Kaypote Elixir 30 mEq bid
   Stock: bottle of liquid labeled 40 mEq per 20 mL

3. Order: Levothroid 100 mcg qd PO
   Stock: scored tablets 0.2 mg

4. Order: ampicillin 2 g IVPB q6h; macrodrip 10 gtt/mL

Drug	Diluent	Time
ampicillin Omnipen Polycillin-N	50 mL (1 gram) NS 100 mL (2 grams)	20–30 min

5. Order: Demerol 75 mg IM stat
   Stock: vial of liquid labeled 100 mg per mL

6. Order: scopolamine 0.5 mg SC stat
   Stock: vial labeled 0.4 mg per mL

7. Order: nafcillin sodium 600 mg IM q6h
   Stock: vial of 2 grams of powder

   Directions for Intramuscular Use: Reconstitute with sterile water for injection, USP, 0.9% sodium chloride injection, USP, or bacteriostatic water for injection, USP (with benzyl alcohol or parabens); add 1.8 mL to the 500-mg vial for 2 mL resulting solution; 3.4 mL to the 1-g vial for 4 mL resulting solution; 6.6 mL to the 2-g vial for 8 mL resulting solution. All reconstituted vials have a concentration of 250 mg per mL. The clear solution should be administered by deep intragluteal injection immediately after reconstitution. The resulting solutions are stable for 3 days at room temperature, 7 days under refrigeration, and 90 days frozen.

8. Order: 1500 mL D5W IV KVO for 24 hr

   a. What tubing will you use?

   b. What is the drop factor?

9. Order: 500 mL D5 ½ NS IV
                 run 75 mL/hr
                 No pump is available

   a. What tubing will you use?

   b. What is the drop factor?

10. Order: heparin 25,000 Units in 250 mL D5W IV
                 infuse 1200 Units per hour
                 An IV pump is available

    What is the drip rate?

Copyright © 2003 Lippincott Williams & Wilkins, *Instructor's Manual and Testbank to Accompany Henke's Med-Math: Dosage Calculation, Preparation, and Administration*, fourth edition, by Susan Buchholz.

■ Med-Math Cumulative Test

Name _____ Date _____

PART 1

Dosage
Directions: Show the arithmetic for dosage answers.

1. Provide the meaning of each of the following abbreviations. Give sample times for those marked with an asterisk. (8 cr)

   a. *bid _____

   b. *q6h _____

   c. OD _____

   d. SL _____

   e. pr _____

   f. *qid _____

   g. *ac _____

   h. *q8h _____

2. Give the equivalent. (10 cr)

   a. 0.3 gm = _____ mg

   b. 0.001 g = _____ mg

   c. 1 oz = _____ mL

   d. 600 mg = _____ g

   e. 200 mcg = _____ mg

   f. 1 dram = _____ cc

   g. 1 tsp = _____ mL

   h. 0.08 mg = _____ mcg

   i. 0.25 mg = _____ mcg

   j. 1 g = _____ mg

3. Order: oral suspension 200 mg PO   (3 cr)
   Stock: 125 mg/5 mL

4. Order: tablets 200 mcg PO   (3 cr)
   Stock: tablets 0.1 mg

5. Order: tablet 0.5 mg PO   (3 cr)
   Stock: 0.25-mg scored tablets

6. Order: liquid 300 mg PO   (3 cr)
   Stock: 250 mg/5 mL

7. Order: Mylanta 30 mL PO   (3 cr)
   Stock: Mylanta double-strength oral suspension

Copyright © 2003 Lippincott Williams & Wilkins, *Instructor's Manual and Testbank to Accompany Henke's Med-Math: Dosage Calculation, Preparation, and Administration,* fourth edition, by Susan Buchholz.

8. Order: liquid 0.125 mg IM   (3 cr)
   Stock: ampule 0.25 mg/2 mL

9. Order: liquid 12 mg SC   (3 cr)
   Stock: liquid 15 mg/mL

10. Order: liquid 50 mg IM   (3 cr)
    Stock: 40 mg/mL liquid

11. Order: ceftazidime 0.3 g IM   (4 cr)
    Stock: vial of powder 1 gram

   Directions: Reconstitution of Single-Dose Vials: For IM injection reconstitute with sterile water for injection according to the following table. Shake well.

Vial Size	Amount of Diluent to be Added	Approximate Available Volume	Approximate Ceftazidime Concentration
500 mg	1.5 mL	1.8 mL	280 mg/mL
1 gram	3.0 mL	3.6 mL	280 mg/mL

Dilute with: _____

Solution: _____

Give: _____

Label: _____

12. Order: Omnipen 250 mg IM   (4cr)
    Stock: vial of 500 mg powder

   Directions: Dissolve 500 mg of powder with 1.8 mL sterile water for injection to make a concentration of 250 mg/mL.

Dilute with: _____

Solution: _____

Give: _____

Label: _____

Copyright © 2003 Lippincott Williams & Wilkins, *Instructor's Manual and Testbank to Accompany Henke's Med-Math: Dosage Calculation, Preparation, and Administration,* fourth edition, by Susan Buchholz.

13. Order: ampicillin 400 mg IM q8h   (4 cr)
    Stock: vial of 1 g powder

Directions: Dissolve 1 gram of powder with 3.4 mL sterile water for injection to make a concentration of 250 mg/mL. The resulting solution must be used within 1 hr after reconstitution.

Dilute with: _____

Solution: _____

Give: _____

Label: _____

14. Order: 500 mL D5W; run 75 mL/hr   (4 cr)
               microtubing is available

15. Order: 1000 mL D5W IV 8 A.M. to 8 P.M.   (4 cr)
               microtubing is available

16. Order: Bactrim 1 ampule in 125 mL D5W qd   (4 cr)
    Stock: 1 ampule
           macrotubing 10 gtt/mL is available

Drug	Diluent	Time
trimethorpim–sulfamethoxazole (Bactrim, Septra)	One 5-mL vial per 75 mL or 125 mL D5W	60–90 min/24 hr

Copyright © 2003 Lippincott Williams & Wilkins, *Instructor's Manual and Testbank to Accompany Henke's Med-Math: Dosage Calculation, Preparation, and Administration,* fourth edition, by Susan Buchholz.

■ Med-Math Cumulative Test

PART II

General Information Related to Drug Administration

17. Match the terms with their explanations. (10 cr)

a. _____ Unit dose	**q.**	Dissolving a powder into a solution.
b. _____ Ampule	**r.**	Glass container with a sealed rubber top.
c. _____ Parenteral	**s.**	Route of administration to skin or mucous membranes.
d. _____ Prefilled cartridge	**t.**	Individually wrapped and labeled drugs.
e. _____ Reconstitution	**u.**	Disklike solid that dissolves in the mouth.
f. _____ Topical	**v.**	Suppository ingredient that melts at room temperature.
g. _____ Transdermal patch	**w.**	General term for an injection route.
h. _____ Vial	**x.**	Adhesive bandage to the skin that gradually releases a drug.
i. _____ Lozenge	**y.**	Small vial, with a needle attached, that fits into a holder.
j. _____ Cocoa butter	**z.**	Glass container that must be broken to obtain the drug.

18. List seven kinds of drug information the nurse needs to know to administer drugs safely. (7 cr)

a. _____

b. _____

c. _____

d. _____

e. _____

f. _____

g. _____

19. List four positive actions the nurse can take to avoid liability (malpractice). (4 cr)

a. _____

b. _____

c. _____

d. _____

Copyright © 2003 Lippincott Williams & Wilkins, *Instructor's Manual and Testbank to Accompany Henke's Med-Math: Dosage Calculation, Preparation, and Administration,* fourth edition, by Susan Buchholz.

20. Name three ethical principles that guide the nurse in administering medications, and give one example of how each principle could be violated by a nurse.   (3 cr)

    a. _____

    b. _____

    c. _____

21. When must medication nurses wash their hands during the administration of drugs?   (3cr)

22. Identify each of these administration procedures as clean (cl) or sterile (st).   (10 cr)

    a. _____ SC injection   f. _____ Nitroglycerin patch

    b. _____ SL tablet   g. _____ Nasogastric route

    c. _____ Vaginal suppository   h. _____ Intradermal

    d. _____ Nose drops   i. _____ Rectal suppository

    e. _____ IM injection   j. _____ Buccal

23. List the four phases of pharmacokinetic action and state where in the body each phase is most likely to occur.   (4 cr)

    a. _____

    b. _____

    c. _____

    d. _____

24. List three reasons for administering medication by injection.   (3 cr)

    a. _____

    b. _____

    c. _____

Copyright © 2003 Lippincott Williams & Wilkins, *Instructor's Manual and Testbank to Accompany Henke's Med-Math: Dosage Calculation, Preparation, and Administration,* fourth edition, by Susan Buchholz.

Test Answers

Chapter 1

ARITHMETIC PRETEST—TEST A

1. a. 17,094
   b. $\frac{2}{3}$
   c. 0.0782
2. a. 16.39
   b. 1.5
   c. 50
3. a. 0.02
   b. 0.8

4. a. $\frac{3}{20}$
   b. $\frac{3}{100}$
5. a. 0.6
   b. 0.4
   c. 0.2
   d. 0.25
6. a. 0.13
   b. 0.23
   c. 0.14

7. a. 3.5
   b. 0.33
   c. 0.725
8. a. $\frac{1}{300}$
   b. 0.009
9. a. 12
   b. 33
   c. 16

ARITHMETIC PRETEST—TEST B

1. a. 37,152
   b. $\frac{3}{40}$
2. a. 142.15
   b. $\frac{11}{4}$ or 2.75
   c. 400
3. a. 0.19
   b. 0.45

4. a. $\frac{1}{250}$
   b. $\frac{1}{4}$
5. a. 0.4
   b. 0.5
   c. 0.46
   d. 0.25
6. a. 0.08
   b. 0.15
   c. 0.22

7. a. 14.6
   b. 0.03
   c. 0.333
8. a. $\frac{1}{400}$
   b. 0.125
9. a. 10
   b. 5
   c. 7.8

Chapter 2

MEDICAL ABBREVIATIONS—TEST A

1. before meals
   7:30 a, 11:30 a, 4:30 p
2. both eyes
3. three times a week
   10 a on Mon, Wed, Fri
4. every four hours
   2 a, 6 a, 10 a, 2 p, 6 p, 10 p
5. subcutaneously
6. by mouth
7. every 12 hr
   6 a, 6 p
8. every day
   10 a
9. three times a day
   10 a, 2 p, 6 a

10. left eye
11. milligram
12. twice a day
    10 a, 6 p
13. milliequivalent
14. right eye
15. four times a day
    10 a, 2 p, 6 a, 10 p
16. every 8 hr
    6 a, 2 p, 10 p
17. every 6 hr
    6 a, 12 noon, 6 p, 12 midnight
18. teaspoon
19. intramuscularly
20. milliliter

Copyright © 2003 Lippincott Williams & Wilkins, *Instructor's Manual and Testbank to Accompany Henke's Med-Math: Dosage Calculation, Preparation, and Administration*, fourth edition, by Susan Buchholz.

MEDICAL ABBREVIATIONS—TEST B

A.
1. d
2. a
3. b
4. f
5. l
6. j
7. k
8. i
9. c
10. h

B.
1. every four hours, 2 a, 6 a, 10 a, 2 p, 6 p, 10 p
2. after meals, 10 a, 2 p, 6 p
3. milliliter
4. twice a week on Mon and Thurs at 10 a
5. teaspoon
6. every other day, 10 a, odd days of the month
7. intramuscularly
8. by mouth
9. milligram
10. sublingual

Chapter 4

MEDICAL EQUIVALENTS—TEST A

1.
a. 250 mg
b. 15 mg
c. 0.05 mg
d. 30 mg
e. 1000 mg
f. 0.001 mg

2.
a. 0.03 g
b. 0.0006 g
c. 0.1 g
d. 0.005 g

3.
a. 250 mcg
b. 125 mcg
c. 500 mcg
d. 100 mcg
e. 10 mcg
f. 1 mcg

4.
a. 8 mL
b. 5 cc
c. 1 mL
d. 1 L
e. 15 cc
f. 1 gtt
g. 30 mL
h. 1000 mL
i. 15 cc

MEDICAL EQUIVALENTS—TEST B

A.
1. 1 g
2. 4000 mcg
3. 0.1 g
4. 1000 mL
5. 5 cc
6. 15 mg
7. 125 mcg
8. 1 mL
9. 200 mg
10. 2.2 lb
11. ½ oz
12. 0.001 g
13. 1000 mg
14. 15 mL
15. 0.01 mg
16. 12 mL
17. 500 mcg
18. 500 cc
19. 0.015 g
20. 0.25 mg

B.
1. a
2. b
3. a
4. a
5. c

Chapter 6

ORAL TABLET PROBLEMS—TEST A

1. 2 tabs
2. ½ tab
3. 2 caps
4. 2 ½ tabs
5. ½ tab
6. 2 caps
7. ½ tab
8. ½ tab
9. 2 tabs
10. ½ tab

ORAL TABLET PROBLEMS—TEST B

1. 2 tabs
2. ½ tab
3. 2 tabs
4. 2 tabs
5. ½ tab
6. ½ tab
7. 2 tabs
8. 2 caps
9. 2 tabs
10. 2 tabs
11. 2 caps
12. 3 caps
13. ½ tab
14. ½ tab
15. 1 tab
16. 1 tab
17. 1 ½ tabs
18. 2 tabs
19. ½ tab
20. 2 ½ tabs

Copyright © 2003 Lippincott Williams & Wilkins, *Instructor's Manual and Testbank to Accompany Henke's Med-Math: Dosage Calculation, Preparation, and Administration*, fourth edition, by Susan Buchholz.

ORAL LIQUID PROBLEMS—TEST A

1. 8 mL	4. 1 oz = 30 mL	7. 10 mL	9. 10 mL
2. 5 mL	5. 5 mL	8. 5 mL	10. 5 mL
3. 20 mL	6. 20 mL		

ORAL LIQUID PROBLEMS—TEST B

1. 8 mL	6. 20 mL	11. 30 mL	16. 15 mL
2. 12 mL	7. 5 mL	12. 15 mL	17. 25 mL
3. 5 mL	8. 8 mL	13. 8 mL	18. 10 mL
4. 5 mL	9. 10 mL	14. 20 mL	19. 6 mL
5. 5 mL	10. 2½ mL	15. 16 mL	20. 5 mL

Chapter 7

INJECTION FROM A LIQUID—TEST A

1. 1 mL	4. 15 Units	7. 0.4 mL	9. 0.25 mL
2. 1.2 mL	5. 1.6 mL	8. 1 mL	10. 0.5 mL
3. 0.53 mL	6. 1.5 mL		

INJECTION FROM A LIQUID—TEST B

1. 1.5 mL	4. 0.5 mL	7. 1 mL	9. 1 mL
2. 1.5 mL	5. 1 mL	8. 1.6 mL	10. 0.67 mL
3. 0.4 mL	6. 0.8 mL		

Chapter 8

INJECTION FROM A POWDER—TEST A

A. 1. Use 250-mg vial
   Add 1.2 mL sterile water
   Solution 208 mg/mL
   Give 1.2 mL
   Label 208 mg/mL; date; initials
2. Use 2-gram vial
   Add sterile water as follows:

Add	Solution and Label	Give
4 mL	1 g per 2.5 mL	1.3 mL
5 mL	1 g per 3.0 mL	1.5 mL
7.2 mL	1 g per 4.0 mL	2.0 mL

3. Use 1-gram vial
   Add 3.0 mL sterile water
   Solution 280 mg/mL
   Give 1.8 mL
   Label 280 mg/mL; date; initials

4. Use 500-mg vial
   Add 1.8 mL sterile water
   Solution 250 mg/mL
   Give 2 mL
   No label; discard vial
5. Use 1-gram vial
   Add 3 mL sterile water
   Solution 300 mg/mL
   Give 1.3 mL
   Label 300 mg/mL; date; initials

Copyright © 2003 Lippincott Williams & Wilkins, *Instructor's Manual and Testbank to Accompany Henke's Med-Math: Dosage Calculation, Preparation, and Administration,* fourth edition, by Susan Buchholz.

INJECTION FROM A POWDER—TEST A

B. 1. Use vial of one million Units
Add 4.6 mL sterile water
Solution 200,000 Units/mL
Give 2 mL
Label 200,000 Units/mL; date; initials
2. Use 1-gram vial
Add 2.5 mL sterile water
Solution 1 gram per 3 mL
Give 1.5 mL
Label 1 g/3 mL; date; initials
3. Use 500-mg ampule
Add 5 mL sterile water
Solution 100 mg/mL
Give 1.5 mL
No label; discard ampule

4. Use 250-mg vial
Add 0.9 mL sterile water
Solution 250 mg/mL
Give 0.6 mL
Label 250 mg/mL; date; initials
5. Use 2-gram vial
Add 4 mL sterile water
Solution 1 g = 2.5 mL
Give 1.3 mL
Label 1 g/2.5 mL; date; initials

INJECTION FROM A POWDER—TEST B

A. 1. Use 1-gram vial
Add 2 mL sterile water
Solution 400 mg/mL
Give 2 mL
Label 400 mg/mL; date; initials
2. Use vial of one million Units
Add 3.6 mL sterile water
Solution 250,000 Units per mL
Give 1 mL
Label 250,000 Units/mL; date; initials
3. Use 500-mg vial
Add 2.0 mL sterile water
Solution 225 mg/mL
Give 1.8 mL
Label 225 mg/mL; date; initials
4. Use 1-gram vial
Add 2 mL sterile water
Solution 1 g/2.6 mL
Give 1.3 mL
Label 1 g = 2.6 mL; date; initials
5. Use 2-gram vial
Add 5.4 mL sterile water and 1.8 mL
lidocaine HCl 0.5%
Solution 250 mg/mL
Give 1.5 mL
Label 250 mg/mL; date; initials
(Directions do not indicate storage)

B. 1. Use 1-gram vial
Add 2.5 mL sterile water
Solution 330 mg/mL
Give 2 mL
Label 330 mg/mL; date; initials
2. Use 1-gram vial
Add 2 mL sterile water
Solution 400 mg/mL
Give 1.5 mL
Label 400 mg/mL; date; initials
3. Use 500-mg vial
Add 2 mL sterile water
Solution 225 mg/mL
Give 2 mL
Label 225 mg/mL; date; initials
4. Use 250-mg ampule
Add 3.8 mL sterile water
Solution 50 mg/mL
Give 2 mL
No label; discard ampule
5. Use 250-mg vial
Add 2 mL sterile water
Solution 125 mg/mL
Give 1.2 mL
Label 125 mg/mL; date; initials

Chapter 9

BASIC IVs—TEST A

1. 63 gtt/min
2. Approximately 7 hr
3. Add 5 mL aminophylline
Set pump at 50 mL/hr
4. 42 gtt/min
5. Microtubing at 50 gtt/min
6. 17 gtt/min
7. Set up at 42 mL/hr
8. Add 8 mL KCl to IV
Use macrotubing at 25 gtt/min
9. No math. Use micro-tubing at 50 mL/hr
10. 33 gtt/min

Copyright © 2003 Lippincott Williams & Wilkins, *Instructor's Manual and Testbank to Accompany Henke's Med-Math: Dosage Calculation, Preparation, and Administration,* fourth edition, by Susan Buchholz.

BASIC IVs—TEST B

1. Approximately 4 hr
2. No math. Set pump at 60 mL/hr
3. 17 gtt/min
4. Add 15 mL KCl to the IV Set IV at 56 gtt/min
5. Use microtubing at 17 gtt/min
6. Add 10 mL aminophylline to the IV No math. Set pump at 75 mL/hr
7. 3920 mL
8. Use 100 mL over 33 gtt/min
9. 42 gtt/min
10. Use microtubing at 21 gtt/min

Chapter 10

SPECIAL IVs—TEST A

1. Set pump 11 mL/hr
2. Set pump 75 mL/hr
3. Set pump 12 mL/hr
4. Set pump 100 mL/hr
5. Set pump 45 mL/hr
6. Set pump 30 mL/hr
7. Set pump 9 mL/hr
8. Set pump 30 mL/hr
9. 1 milliunit/min = 60 milliunits/hr
    Set pump 3 mL/h4
10. a. Yes (297.5 = 300)
    b. 21 mL/hr

SPECIAL IVs—TEST B

1. Set pump 14 mL/hr
2. Set pump 30 mL/hr
3. Set pump 10 mL/hr
4. Set pump 60 mL/hr
5. Set pump 8 mL/hr
6. Set pump 18 mL/hr
7. Set pump 5 mL/hr
8. 0.5 mg/min = 30 mg/hr Set pump 30 mL/hr
9. Set pump 60 mL/hr
10. a. Yes
    b. 42 mL/hr

Chapter 11

DOSAGE PROBLEMS FOR INFANTS AND CHILDREN—TEST A

1. a. Range 300 mg/kg to 600 mg/kg
    Dose is safe (300 mg/day)
   b. 4 mL
2. a. Range 70 mg/day to 140 mg/day
    Dose is safe (105 mg)
   b. 3.5 mL
3. 1 mL
4. 40 mg/kg/day = 175 mg PO q8h
    40 mg/kg/day × 4.3 kg = 172 mg per day
    Dose of 175 mg q8h is excessive
    Check with the physician. Do not administer
5. 22 lb = 10 kg
   a. Safe range is 30–50 mg. Dose is safe
   b. 1 mL
6. a. 50,000 Units/kg × 48 kg = 2.4 million Units
    Dose is safe
   b. 4 mL IM. Split the dose. Give 2 mL in each buttock
7. a. 2.5 mg/kg q12h × 4 kg = 10 per dose.
    Dose is safe
   b. Gentamycin pediatric is 10 mg/mL delivery.
    Draw up 1 mL. Volume for IVPB is 1 mg/mL.
    Total volume is 1 mL gentamycin plus 9 mL diluent
8. a. 5 mL KCl
   b. Add 35 cc of IV to the Buretrol from the reservoir
   c. Set the pump for 35 mL/hr
9. a. 1.9 mL
   b. 17 gtt per min
10. a. Child weighs 6.8 kg
    44 mg × 6.8 kg = 299.2 mg in divided doses
    100 mg q8h is a safe dose
    b. Add 1.2 mL vancomycin to the Buretrol. Run in D5 ⅓ NS to reach 20 mL.
    c. Set the pump for 40 mL/hr (you want 20 mL in 30 min, but the pump delivers mL/hr; the patient will receive 20 mL in 30 min)

Copyright © 2003 Lippincott Williams & Wilkins, *Instructor's Manual and Testbank to Accompany Henke's Med-Math: Dosage Calculation, Preparation, and Administration*, fourth edition, by Susan Buchholz.

DOSAGE PROBLEMS FOR INFANTS AND CHILDREN—TEST B

1. **a.** 41 kg × 15 mg = 615 mg/day. Dose is safe
   b. One 400-mg tab
   Two 100-mg tabs
2. 0.9 mL
3. **a.** 8.4 × 10 mg = 84 mg. Dose is safe
   b. 2.4 mL
4. **a.** 4 mg/kg q6h = 4 × 18.9 × 4 = 302.4 mg
   Do not exceed 24 mg/kg/day = 18.9 × 24 mg = 453.6 mg maximum
   Dose is safe
   b. 23.4 mL
5. **a.** Range is 420 mg/kg to 840 mg/kg/day
   Dose is safe (210 mg × 3 doses = 630 mg/day)
   b. Cefuroxime is 90 mg/mL. Draw up 2.3 mL. Add to the Buretrol. Fill up to 20 mL with D5 ⅓ NS. Set the pump for 40 mL/hr (you want 20 mL over 30 min, but the pump delivers mL/hr; the patient will receive 20 mL over 30 min)
6. **a.** 50 mg × 9 kg = 450 mg/day
   Dose is safe (150 mg × 3 doses = 450 mg)
   b. 0.7 mL

7. **a.** 5 mg × 12 kg = 60 mg/day
   Dose is safe (15 mg × 4 doses = 60 mg)
   b. 0.3 mL
8. **a.** Range is 114 mg/day to 142.5 mg/day
   Dose is safe (40 mg × 3 doses = 120 mg)
   b. 1 mL. Use a Buretrol. Add 1 mL tobramycin; add D5 ⅓ NS from the reservoir to make 20 cc. Set the pump for 40 mL/hr because it delivers mL/hr. The patient will receive 20 mL in 30 min
9. **a.** 75 mg/kg/day = 360 mg/day is a safe dose
   210 mg × 3 = 630 mg/day
   Dose is beyond the safe range. Check with the physician
   b. Do not administer
10. **a.** Dose is safe. Literature states 1.2 MU q month is a single dose
    b. 2 mL

Cumulative Dosage Test

TEST A

1. 2 tabs
2. 10 mL
3. ½ tab
4. Use vial of 1 million Units
   Add 9.6 mL DW
   Solution 100,000 Units/mL
   Give 1.5 mL
   Label 100,000 Units/mL; date; initials
5. 1 mL

6. 42 gtt/min
7. Use NPH insulin U 100/mL
   Use lo dose insulin syringe
   Draw up 30 Units
8. **a.** 25 gtt/min
   b. 4 hr
9. 0.5 mL
10. 15 mL/hr

TEST B

1. 5 mL
2. 15 mL
3. ½ tab
4. 33 gtt/min
5. 0.8 mL
6. 1.3 mL
7. Use 2-gram vial
   Add 6.6 mL sterile water
   Solution 250 mg/mL
   Give 2.4 mL
   Label 250 mg/mL; date; initials

8. **a.** Microdrip tubing
   b. 63 gtt/min
9. **a.** Microtubing
   b. 75 gtt/min
10. Set pump at 12 mL/hr

Copyright © 2003 Lippincott Williams & Wilkins, *Instructor's Manual and Testbank to Accompany Henke's Med-Math: Dosage Calculation, Preparation, and Administration,* fourth edition, by Susan Buchholz.

Med-Math Cumulative Test

PART I

1. **a.** Twice a day
      10 a, 6 p
   b. Every 6 hr
      6 a, 12 noon, 6 p, 12 midnight
   c. Right eye
   d. Sublingual
   e. By rectum
   f. Four times a day
      10 a, 2 p, 6 p, 10 p
   g. Before meals
      7:30 a, 11:30 a, 4:30 p
   h. Every 8 hr
      6 a, 2 p, 10 p

2. **a.** 300 mg   **f.** 4 cc
   b. 1 mg   **g.** 5 mL
   c. 30 mL   **h.** 80 mcg
   d. 0.6 g   **i.** 250 mcg
   e. 0.2 mg   **j.** 1000 mg

3. 8 mL
4. 2 tabs
5. 2 tabs
6. 6 mL
7. 15 mL (double strength)
8. 1 mL

9. 0.8 mL
10. 1.3 mL
11. Use 1-gram vial
    Add 3 mL sterile water
    Solution 280 mg/mL
    Give 1.1 mL
    Label 290 mg/mL; date; initials
12. Use 500-mg vial
    Add 1.8 mL sterile water
    Solution 250 mg/mL
    Give 1 mL
    Label 250 mg/mL; date; initials
13. Use 1-gram vial
    Add 3.4 mL sterile water
    Solution 250 mg/mL
    Give 1.6 mL
    No label. Discard. Use within 1 hr
14. No math. Use microtubing
    75 gtt/min
15. Use microtubing
    83 gtt/min
16. 60 min—use 21 gtt/min
    90 min—use 14 gtt/min

Copyright © 2003 Lippincott Williams & Wilkins, *Instructor's Manual and Testbank to Accompany Henke's Med-Math: Dosage Calculation, Preparation, and Administration,* fourth edition, by Susan Buchholz.

PART II

17. a. t   f. s
    b. z   g. x
    c. w   h. r
    d. y   i. u
    e. q   j. v

18. Trade and generic names; drug class; pregnancy category; dosage and route; action; uses; side and adverse effects; contraindications; precautions; interactions; incompatibilities; nursing implications

19. Know and follow institutional policies; look up drugs that are unfamiliar; do not leave medications at the bedside; chart carefully; listen and act when the patient says, "I never took that before"; double check a dose that seems high; label any powder you dilute and any IV bag you use; seek advice from competent professionals; do not give drugs poured by another nurse; keep drug knowledge current; attend CE programs; update skills

20. Autonomy—force a patient to take a medication that he has refused
    Truthfulness—lying to a patient about the effects of a drug
    Beneficence—not providing full disclosure in obtaining permission
    Nonmaleficience—neglect to report a colleague abusing drugs
    Confidentiality—talking about a patient in the cafeteria within listening distance of others
    Justice—failing to give the right drug in the right dose to the right patient at the right time

21. Hands must be washed before preparing medications and after administering medications to each patient. Hands must be washed after removing gloves, gowns, masks, or goggles, and before leaving the room of any patient for whom they are used. Hands must be washed immediately when soiled with patient blood or bodily fluid. Hands must be washed when handling equipment soiled with blood or bodily fluids.

22. a. st   f. cl
    b. cl   g. cl
    c. cl   h. st
    d. cl   i. cl
    e. st   j. cl

23. a. Absorption—mainly through small intestinal villi
    b. Distribution—blood stream
    c. Biostransformation—mainly liver
    d. Excretion—mainly kidney

24. The drug cannot be given orally; it is necessary to obtain a rapid systemic effect; the drug would be rendered ineffective or destroyed by the oral route

Copyright © 2003 Lippincott Williams & Wilkins, *Instructor's Manual and Testbank to Accompany Henke's Med-Math: Dosage Calculation, Preparation, and Administration,* fourth edition, by Susan Buchholz.

Test Your Clinical Savvy Answers

Test Your Clinical Savvy was designed to suggest clinical situations where dosage calculations may not have a "right or wrong" solution. Certainly the math involved in calculations is either correct or incorrect. However, to promote critical thinking, these scenarios are meant to get you to think about several possibilities or options in a clinical setting. Sometimes more information is needed to answer these problems. With that in mind, here are some possible "answers" to Test Your Clinical Savvy.

■ Chapter 7

A. Could you use a 3-mL syringe to draw up insulin? If so, how is this done and what would be the precautions?
   - It would be dangerous to use a larger syringe such as the 3-mL to draw up insulin, because the markings for the tenths of a cc are so small. However, it would be possible, especially if the dose is large enough. The nurse should remember that 100 units of insulin equals 1 cc. In addition, a double-check of the dose and the syringe amount with another nurse should be done.

B. Could a 5-mL syringe be used to draw up insulin?
   - It would be even more dangerous to use a 5-mL syringe. The same answer would apply as above, in that if it is a large enough dose (eg, 50 units of insulin), then you could use a large syringe and draw up 0.5 cc of insulin.

C. What would be the danger in using either of these syringes?
   - Inaccurate dose—either too little or too much of the insulin.

D. What amount of insulin would be safe to draw up in either a 3-mL or 5-mL syringe (or neither)?
   - Using safety as the rule, neither syringe should be used. Using practicality, probably no less than 0.5 cc of insulin.

E. Even if a 1-mL syringe were available, what would be the precautions in using a non-insulin syringe?
   - Careful calculation of the dose of insulin, correct type of insulin, correct amount of insulin drawn up in the syringe, double-checking the dose and syringe amount with another nurse, and use of correct needle.

Copyright © 2003 Lippincott Williams & Wilkins, *Instructor's Manual and Testbank to Accompany Henke's Med-Math: Dosage Calculation, Preparation, and Administration,* fourth edition, by Susan Buchholz.

■ Chapter 8

A. What should you do to ensure that no mistakes are made for the initial dosing and for subsequent dosing of penicillin?

- Read the vial carefully to ensure the correct directions are followed for initial reconstitution. Clarify with another nurse or the pharmacist if there are any questions. Utilize the *PDR* to clarify reconstitution directions.
- Clearly label the vial with date, time, initials, and concentration after reconstitution (eg, 1,000,000 units = 1 mL). Recording the concentration after reconstitution on the medication record is suggested.

B. What is the danger in administering too much of any drug?

- Cardiac arrest, shock, anaphylaxis, respiratory arrest or difficulty, mild or moderate allergic reaction, organ damage.

C. What is the danger in administering too much penicillin and/or potassium?

- Possibilities as in answer B. Cardiac arrest, especially from too much potassium. Possible anaphylaxis from too much penicillin.

■ Chapter 10

A. Why would an infusion pump be needed with these medications?

- All of these drugs have major effects on the body. These drugs also have adverse effects that can be serious or life-threatening. These medications also require blood levels to monitor the desired therapeutic levels. Using an infusion pump carefully regulates the amount of drug the patient is receiving.

B. Why would medications that are based on body weight require the use of a pump? Why would medications based on BSA require an infusion pump?

- Medications based on body weight or BSA require an exact dosing, which only an infusion pump can provide.

C. Can any of these medications be regulated with standard roller clamp tubing? What would be the advantage? What would be the contraindications?

- From a safety perspective, no. However, one clinical situation encountered by the author was a critical care patient who needed an MRI. Because infusion pumps are made of metal and no metal can be present with an MRI, the IV infusions were regulated by a standard roller clamp. Microdrip tubing must be used if this is the situation. Careful calculation of the dose and careful regulation must be done. Use of a roller clamp for regulation can be very inaccurate, especially with any position changes of the patient. Contraindications would be using roller clamp regulation with a critically ill patient and with vasoactive medications. Also, certain medications such as the ones mentioned in this scenario should use infusion pumps.

Copyright © 2003 Lippincott Williams & Wilkins, *Instructor's Manual and Testbank to Accompany Henke's Med-Math: Dosage Calculation, Preparation, and Administration,* fourth edition, by Susan Buchholz.

▪ Chapter 11

A. What could you do to help her take the medication? Are there other alternatives you could use in regards to the medication? What would you suggest to the family to promote easier compliance?

- Mix the medication with liquid or soft food (applesauce, gelatin, ice cream); make sure the drug is diluted in the smallest amount of liquid or food so that the child receives the full dose. See if the oral medication comes in liquid or chewable form; give the child a choice of these. Offering popsicles or ice chips helps numb the taste buds and promote cooperation. Nurses and parents can reinforce and reassure children that the drug is to help them feel better and keep them healthy. Assess the child and family relationship; would the child be more compliant with or without the parents present? Reward rather than punishment should be utilized.

B. Besides reducing the possibility of fluid overload, what are some other reasons IV infusion pumps are used with children?

- Careful monitoring of drug dosage (drug dosage in children is more exact and based on weight); infusion pumps will help monitor possible infiltration, air bubbles/possible air embolism, and occlusion.

C. Another patient, 11-year-old Sean McBrady, is unable to swallow pills. What are some alternatives to the medication? What would you suggest to the family and patient to promote easier administration?

- See whether a liquid or chewable form of the medication is available. See whether the pills can be crushed and mixed in a liquid or soft food. Work on techniques of swallowing pills: place the pill on the back of the tongue and immediately drink fluid; break the pill into smaller amounts and administer; place the pill in the mouth and immediately drink fluid; ask family members or other health care personnel for any suggestions.

▪ Chapter 12

Caveat: The following questions are very difficult to answer, even for experienced nurses. Every specific clinical situation and every specific patient must be considered.

A. What is your responsibility as a nurse ethically when administering this drug?

- A nurse should know about the drug, side effects, correct dosage, and indications for the drug. If there is a research trial, the nurse should be aware of the trial and whether there is a referral person or phone number. In a hospital setting, the nurse should be familiar with policies regarding the role of the nurse with investigational drugs. The nurse should serve as the patient's advocate in working with patients involved in drug studies. Finally, the nurse should not violate ethical principles.

B. What is an appropriate response if the patient asks, "Is it safe to take this drug?" What should you do if the patient refuses to take the drug?

Copyright © 2003 Lippincott Williams & Wilkins, *Instructor's Manual and Testbank to Accompany Henke's Med-Math: Dosage Calculation, Preparation, and Administration,* fourth edition, by Susan Buchholz.

- Some of the responsibilities in answer A also apply. Before administering the drug, the nurse should consult with any support personnel involved in the research study as to possible responses to this question. Nurses could also discuss possible responses to this question with other nurses. If a patient refuses to take the medication, then a referral should be made to the research study personnel or physician. Thorough documentation of the refusal should be done.

C. You are in agreement with the patient that he or she should not take the experimental drug. What are your ethical responsibilities? What are your legal responsibilities?

- Ethically, the nurse is bound by several principles. Beneficence or do good, and non-maleficence or do no harm, would suggest that the nurse not administer the drug. Also, autonomy means the patient has the right to refuse the drug. Veracity or truthfulness would suggest that the nurse be honest and tell the patient that the nurse agrees with him or her. However, all these principles could also be used to insist the patient take the drug so that it would "do good for them" and not inflict the nurse's opinion or belief on the patient. Legally, a patient can refuse the drug and the nurse cannot force the drug upon a patient. Again, thorough documentation should be completed.

▪ Chapter 13

A. When would the deltoid muscle be preferable or used over either of these sites? What are the contraindications for using the deltoid muscle?

- If there are any contraindications for using the gluteus maximus or vastus lateralis (eg, limb injury, ischemia, recent surgery), then the deltoid may be used. Some IM injections, especially tetanus, are meant to be given in the deltoid. Contraindications include age (the deltoid site is not used in infants or children), injecting more than 1 mL of fluid, any injury, surgery (mastectomy), and pre-existing conditions (renal shunts) of the upper extremities. Some literature recommends not giving IM injections in limbs affected by a CVA.

B. The client requests the injection in the deltoid. What is your response in light of the recommended site in the drug literature?

- All things mentioned in answer A should be considered. Consult with a pharmacist, physician, or health care practitioner about the possibility of a deltoid injection despite the literature recommendation. Client teaching and explanation should be given if another site is still indicated.

Copyright © 2003 Lippincott Williams & Wilkins, *Instructor's Manual and Testbank to Accompany Henke's Med-Math: Dosage Calculation, Preparation, and Administration,* fourth edition, by Susan Buchholz.

C. If a patient is bedridden, which site would you choose for an IM injection and why?

- Some literature suggests the gluteus maximus (dorsogluteal) site has a high rate of potential injury because of its position near the sciatic nerve. Other literature recommends this site because of the larger muscle mass. Basics for any IM injection include good visualization of the site, careful mapping of the site using recommended landmarks, and exposing the site completely. For a bedridden patient, these basics apply. It may be difficult to visualize the dorsogluteal site in a bedridden patient. If the patient can be put into a prone position or turned on the side completely with knees flexed, then this site can be used. Otherwise, the vastus lateralis site can be used if there are no contraindications.

D. Why are gloves necessary when giving IM injections, since you are not actually touching the injection site?

- There is always a possibility that bleeding may occur from the injection site or that other body fluids may be present.

Copyright © 2003 Lippincott Williams & Wilkins, *Instructor's Manual and Testbank to Accompany Henke's Med-Math: Dosage Calculation, Preparation, and Administration,* fourth edition, by Susan Buchholz.

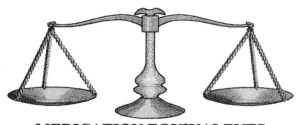

MEDICATION EQUIVALENTS

1 mg	=	1000 mcg
1 Gram (g)	=	1000 mg
1 Kg	=	1000 g
1 Liter	=	1000 mL (cc)
1 Gram (g)	=	gr 15 (approx)
gr i	=	60 mg (approx)
i dram	=	4 mL
i ounce	=	30 mL
1 tsp	=	5 mL
1 tbs	=	15 mL
2.2 lb	=	1 Kg
1 inch	=	2.54 cm

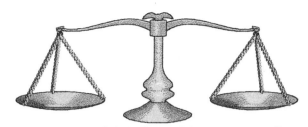

MEDICATION EQUIVALENTS

1 mg	=	1000 mcg
1 Gram (g)	=	1000 mg
1 Kg	=	1000 g
1 Liter	=	1000 mL (cc)
1 Gram (g)	=	gr 15 (approx)
gr i	=	60 mg (approx)
i dram	=	4 mL
i ounce	=	30 mL
1 tsp	=	5 mL
1 tbs	=	15 mL
2.2 lb	=	1 Kg
1 inch	=	2.54 cm

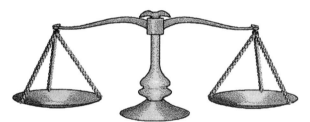

MEDICATION EQUIVALENTS

1 mg	=	1000 mcg
1 Gram (g)	=	1000 mg
1 Kg	=	1000 g
1 Liter	=	1000 mL (cc)
1 Gram (g)	=	gr 15 (approx)
gr i	=	60 mg (approx)
i dram	=	4 mL
i ounce	=	30 mL
1 tsp	=	5 mL
1 tbs	=	15 mL
2.2 lb	=	1 Kg
1 inch	=	2.54 cm

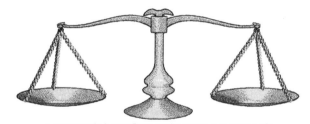

MEDICATION EQUIVALENTS

1 mg	=	1000 mcg
1 Gram (g)	=	1000 mg
1 Kg	=	1000 g
1 Liter	=	1000 mL (cc)
1 Gram (g)	=	gr 15 (approx)
gr i	=	60 mg (approx)
i dram	=	4 mL
i ounce	=	30 mL
1 tsp	=	5 mL
1 tbs	=	15 mL
2.2 lb	=	1 Kg
1 inch	=	2.54 cm

FIVE RIGHTS
Patient
Drug
Dose
Route
Time

CHECK
Patient's allergies

LABEL CHECKS
When reaching for the medication
Immediately before opening
When replacing the medication

FIVE RIGHTS
Patient
Drug
Dose
Route
Time

CHECK
Patient's allergies

LABEL CHECKS
When reaching for the medication
Immediately before opening
When replacing the medication

FIVE RIGHTS
Patient
Drug
Dose
Route
Time

CHECK
Patient's allergies

LABEL CHECKS
When reaching for the medication
Immediately before opening
When replacing the medication

FIVE RIGHTS
Patient
Drug
Dose
Route
Time

CHECK
Patient's allergies

LABEL CHECKS
When reaching for the medication
Immediately before opening
When replacing the medication